Dental Trauma - Expert Strategies

Edited by Betsy Joseph and Sukumaran Anil

Published in London, United Kingdom

Dental Trauma - Expert Strategies
http://dx.doi.org/10.5772/intechopen.1001760
Edited by Betsy Joseph and Sukumaran Anil

Contributors
Amina Gharibi, Anil Sukumaran, Betsy Joseph, Elena Furman, Fernanda Gabriela Carmona Barreto, Genesis Aileen Gordillo-Renteria, Jamila Kissa, Jessika Yesenia Rodriguez Cumbicus, Kumari Abhilasha, Lorena Alexandra Gonzalez Campoverde, Lorenzo Puebla Ramos, María Isabel Cabrera Padrón, Nadia Khlil, Ronald Roossevelt Ramos Montiel, Samia Belfellah, Sergio Oscar Palmas, Sihame Chemlali, Tak On Ryan Tse

First published in London, United Kingdom, 2025 by IntechOpen
IntechOpen is the global imprint of INTECHOPEN LIMITED, registered in England and Wales, registration number: 11086078, 167-169 Great Portland Street, London, W1W 5PF, United Kingdom

For EU product safety concerns: IN TECH d.o.o., Prolaz Marije Krucifikse Kozulić 3, 51000 Rijeka, Croatia, info@intechopen.com or visit our website at intechopen.com.

British Library Cataloguing-in-Publication Data
A catalogue record for this book is available from the British Library

Dental Trauma - Expert Strategies
Edited by Betsy Joseph and Sukumaran Anil
p. cm.

This title is part of the Dentistry Book Series, Volume 22
Topic: Prosthodontics and Implant Dentistry
Series Editor: Sergio Alexandre Gehrke
Topic Editor: Wen Lin Chai
Associate Topic Editor: Ghee Seong Lim

Print ISBN 978-0-85466-396-5
Online ISBN 978-0-85466-395-8
eBook (PDF) ISBN 978-0-85466-544-0
ISSN 2631-6218

IntechOpen Book Series

Dentistry

Volume 22

Aims and Scope of the Series

This book series will offer a comprehensive overview of recent research trends as well as clinical applications within different specialties of dentistry. Topics will include overviews of the health of the oral cavity, from prevention and care to different treatments for the rehabilitation of problems that may affect the organs and/or tissues present. The different areas of dentistry will be explored, with the aim of disseminating knowledge and providing readers with new tools for the comprehensive treatment of their patients with greater safety and with current techniques. Ongoing issues, recent advances, and future diagnostic approaches and therapeutic strategies will also be discussed. This series of books will focus on various aspects of the properties and results obtained by the various treatments available, whether preventive or curative.

Meet the Series Editor

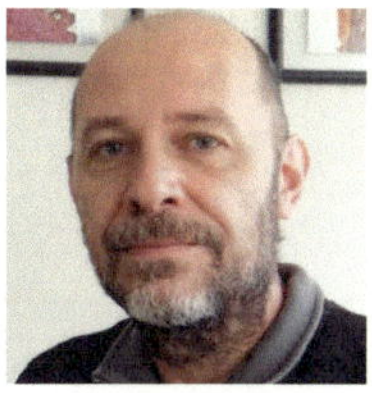

Dr. Sergio Alexandre Gehrke is a doctorate holder in two fields. The first is a Ph.D. in Cellular and Molecular Biology from the Pontificia Catholic University, Porto Alegre, Brazil, in 2010 and the other is an International Ph.D. in Bioengineering from the Universidad Miguel Hernandez, Elche/Alicante, Spain, obtained in 2020. In 2018, he completed a postdoctoral fellowship in Materials Engineering in the NUCLEMAT of the Pontificia Catholic University, Porto Alegre, Brazil. He is currently the Director of the Postgraduate Program in Implantology of the Bioface/UCAM/PgO (Montevideo, Uruguay), Director of the Cathedra of Biotechnology of the Catholic University of Murcia (Murcia, Spain), an Extraordinary Full Professor of the Catholic University of Murcia (Murcia, Spain) as well as the Director of the private center of research Biotecnos – Technology and Science (Montevideo, Uruguay). Applied biomaterials, cellular and molecular biology, and dental implants are among his research interests. He has published several original papers in renowned journals. In addition, he is also a Collaborating Professor in several Postgraduate programs at different universities all over the world.

Meet the Volume Editors

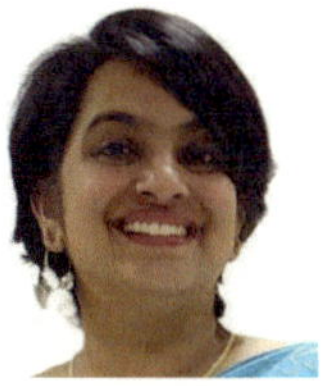

Prof. Betsy Joseph is a renowned periodontist and researcher with expertise in clinical practice, dental education, and scientific research. She is a professor at Saveetha Dental College and a researcher at the University of Helsinki. Her research interests include photodynamic therapy, low-level light therapy, oral pathologies, periodontal diseases, and salivary diagnostics. Prof. Joseph has published extensively, authored book chapters, and conducted funded research projects. She is affiliated with several prestigious organizations and actively contributes to dental research and education.

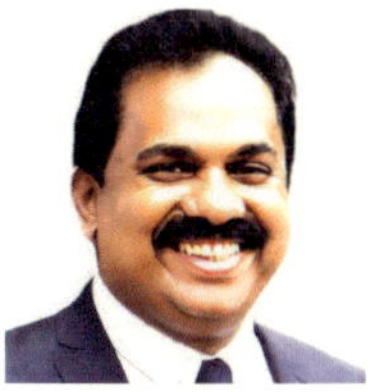

Prof. Anil Sukumaran is a distinguished dental professional and academician with over 36 years of experience. He is a senior consultant professor and chairman of Hospital Research at Hamad Medical Corporation, Qatar. He earned his Ph.D. in dentistry from the University of Hong Kong and has received numerous fellowships, including from the Royal College of Pathologists and the Pierre Fauchard Academy. Prof. Sukumaran has made significant contributions to dental research and education, publishing over 400 research papers and mentoring students globally. He has held key positions at prestigious institutions like King Saud University, where he established a medical research facility. His expertise lies in biomaterials, dentistry, and oral health.

Contents

Preface **XIII**

Chapter 1 **1**
Contemporary Advances in Diagnosis, Management, and Prevention of Traumatic Dental Injuries
by Anil Sukumaran and Betsy Joseph

Chapter 2 **27**
Vertical Root Fracture: The Diagnostic Challenge
by Samia Belfellah, Amina Gharibi, Sihame Chemlali, Nadia Khlil and Jamila Kissa

Chapter 3 **41**
Dental Trauma and Association with Periodontium
by Kumari Abhilasha

Chapter 4 **63**
Association between Dental Trauma and Periodontal Disease
by Elena Furman

Chapter 5 **77**
"Socket Oriented" Tooth Repositioning in Traumatic Dental Injuries
by Tak On Ryan Tse

Chapter 6 **95**
Effectiveness of Oral Splints in Temporomandibular Disorders
by Ronald Roossevelt Ramos-Montiel, Genesis Aileen Gordillo-Renteria, Lorenzo Puebla-Ramos, Sergio Oscar-Palmas, Lorena Alexandra Gonzalez-Campoverde, María Isabel Cabrera-Padrón, Jessika Yesenia Rodriguez-Cumbicus and Fernanda Gabriela Carmona-Barreto

Preface

Dental trauma remains one of the most challenging aspects of contemporary dental practice, demanding immediate clinical expertise and a profound understanding of long-term implications for patient care. This edited volume, *Dental Trauma – Expert Strategies*, presents a comprehensive exploration of current concepts, diagnostic methodologies, and treatment approaches that define modern traumatic dental injury management. The increasing prevalence of dental trauma, coupled with evolving diagnostic technologies and treatment modalities, necessitates a thorough understanding of evidence-based approaches to patient care. This book addresses this need through a carefully structured progression of topics, beginning with fundamental concepts and advancing to specialized treatment strategies.

The opening chapter, "Contemporary Advances in Diagnosis, Management, and Prevention of Traumatic Dental Injuries", establishes the foundational framework necessary for understanding modern trauma management. It introduces current diagnostic protocols, treatment planning considerations, and preventive strategies that form the backbone of clinical decision-making in trauma cases. Building on these foundations, the second chapter "Vertical Root Fracture: The Diagnostic Challenge", addresses one of the most challenging diagnostic scenarios in dental trauma: vertical root fractures. This complex condition often presents diagnostic difficulties that can significantly impact treatment outcomes. The chapter provides detailed insights into advanced diagnostic approaches and interpretation strategies that enhance clinical accuracy.

The third and fourth chapters comprehensively examine the crucial relationship between dental trauma and periodontal health. "Dental Trauma and Association with Periodontium", explores the immediate impact of traumatic injuries on periodontal tissues. At the same time, "Association between Dental Trauma and Periodontal Disease" extends this understanding to long-term implications. Together, these chapters bridge the gap between acute trauma management and chronic disease progression, offering valuable insights into the complex interplay between traumatic injuries and periodontal health. The fifth chapter introduces an innovative approach to trauma management through " "Socket Oriented" Tooth Repositioning in Traumatic Dental Injuries". This technique represents a significant advancement in trauma care, offering predictable outcomes in challenging cases. The chapter provides detailed protocols and clinical considerations that enable practitioners to implement this approach effectively. The final chapter examines the "Effectiveness of Oral Splints in Temporomandibular Disorders", completing the volume's progression from diagnosis to treatment. This evidence-based assessment of splint therapy offers practical insights into managing the broader implications of dental trauma, particularly its impact on temporomandibular function.

We sincerely thank all contributing authors whose expertise and dedication have made this comprehensive volume possible. Their commitment to advancing the field of dental traumatology is evident in the depth and quality of their contributions. Special thanks are due to our editorial assistant, who provided invaluable support throughout the development of this work.

We hope this book will serve as both a practical guide for clinicians and a stimulus for further research in dental trauma. The strategies and insights presented here reflect current best practices while pointing toward future developments in trauma management.

Betsy Joseph
Professor,
Saveetha Institute of Medical and Technical Sciences,
Chennai, India

Anil Sukumaran
Professor,
Hamad Medical Corporation,
Doha, Qatar

Chapter 1

Contemporary Advances in Diagnosis, Management, and Prevention of Traumatic Dental Injuries

Anil Sukumaran and Betsy Joseph

Abstract

Traumatic dental injuries (TDIs) represent a significant global healthcare challenge, affecting different age groups and socioeconomic strata. This comprehensive chapter presents contemporary advances in diagnosing, managing, and preventing TDIs, integrating evidence-based approaches with emerging technologies and biological interventions. The text systematically addresses the multifaceted nature of dental trauma, from immediate emergency response to long-term rehabilitation, while considering the broader implications for healthcare systems and society. Recent developments in diagnostic technologies, including artificial intelligence-assisted imaging and advanced assessment tools, have transformed the initial evaluation of dental trauma. The chapter explores innovative treatment modalities, encompassing regenerative endodontics, stem cell applications, and computer-guided interventions alongside traditional approaches. Particular emphasis is placed on integrating digital workflows, teledentistry applications, and minimally invasive techniques that have revolutionized trauma management. The text critically examines the socioeconomic impact of TDI, including direct and indirect costs, quality of life considerations, and healthcare resource allocation. Special attention is given to age-specific management protocols, medically compromised patients, and legal-ethical considerations. The chapter concludes with an analysis of emerging technologies and future directions in dental traumatology, providing a framework for continued advancement.

Keywords: traumatic dental injuries, dental trauma management, regenerative endodontics, digital dentistry, teledentistry, artificial intelligence in dentistry, minimally invasive dentistry, emergency dental care, dental imaging technologies

1. Introduction

Traumatic dental injuries (TDIs) represent one of the most significant challenges in contemporary dental practice, constituting a major public health concern with far-reaching implications for patient care, healthcare systems, and society at large. The management of TDIs has evolved significantly in recent years, driven by technological advancement, improved understanding of wound healing biology, and the development of innovative treatment modalities [1]. The impact of TDIs extends beyond immediate physical injury, encompassing psychological, functional, and esthetic consequences that can significantly affect a patient's quality of life. Recent epidemiological data indicates that TDIs affect approximately one-third of the global population at some point, with peak incidence occurring during childhood and adolescence [2]. This high prevalence and the potential for long-term complications underscores the importance of effective management strategies.

This chapter comprehensively examines contemporary approaches to TDI management, incorporating the latest evidence-based protocols and innovative technologies. Key areas of focus include:

1. Advanced diagnostic methodologies, including artificial intelligence-assisted imaging and novel assessment tools.

2. Emergency management protocols incorporating teledentistry and digital documentation systems.

3. Regenerative approaches utilizing stem cell therapy and bioactive materials.

4. Minimally invasive surgical techniques and computer-aided interventions.

5. Prevention strategies and risk management protocols.

6. Long-term follow-up and complication management.

The integration of these various elements represents a paradigm shift in TDI management, moving from traditional reactive approaches to more predictable, biology-based interventions. This chapter aims to provide clinicians with a thorough understanding of current best practices while highlighting emerging technologies and future directions in dental traumatology.

2. Epidemiology of traumatic dental injuries (TDI)

Traumatic dental injuries (TDI) represent a significant public health challenge that affects populations worldwide, crossing age groups, socioeconomic strata, and geographic boundaries. The impact of these injuries extends beyond immediate dental health concerns, encompassing psychological, social, and economic implications for individuals, families, and healthcare systems [3]. Understanding TDI's epidemiological patterns, risk factors, and socioeconomic burden is crucial for developing effective prevention strategies and optimizing treatment protocols [4].

2.1 Global prevalence and incidence

The global burden of traumatic dental injuries presents a complex epidemiological picture, with varying prevalence rates reported across different regions and populations. Studies indicate that approximately one-third of preschool children, one-fourth of school-age children, and nearly one-third of adults have experienced trauma to their permanent dentition [5, 6]. These statistics underscore the pervasive nature of dental trauma as a public health concern. In developed nations, the prevalence of TDI in permanent teeth ranges from 20 to 30% among children, with peak incidence occurring between ages 8 and 12 years. This age-related pattern corresponds with developmental stages when children become physically active and engage in sports and recreational activities [7]. Urban populations typically show higher prevalence rates than rural areas, possibly due to differences in lifestyle factors and environmental hazards [8].

The distribution of TDI varies significantly across geographical regions. Studies from South America report prevalence rates as high as 58% in some urban populations, while European studies generally indicate lower rates, ranging from 15 to 25% [9]. Asian countries demonstrate considerable variation, with rates between 16 and 40% depending on the region and study methodology. These disparities may reflect differences in cultural practices, environmental factors, and access to preventive dental care [10].

Gender distribution patterns show a consistent trend across most studies, with males experiencing a higher frequency of dental trauma compared to females, particularly during childhood and adolescence. This disparity is often attributed to males' more significant participation in contact sports and risk-taking behaviors [11]. However, recent studies suggest this gender gap may be narrowing in some populations, possibly reflecting changing social norms and increased female participation in sports activities. The pattern of injury varies with age and dentition type. Primary dentition injuries most commonly occur between ages 2 and 4, corresponding to young children developing motor skills [12]. In permanent dentition, peak incidence occurs during school years, with maxillary central incisors being the most frequently affected teeth, accounting for approximately 80% of all dental injuries in both dentitions [13].

2.2 Risk factors and common causes of traumatic dental injuries

The etiology of traumatic dental injuries (TDI) is multifactorial, encompassing physical, behavioral, and environmental risk factors (**Table 1**). Understanding these factors is crucial for developing targeted prevention strategies and identifying high-risk populations requiring special attention [14].

2.3 Classification of traumatic dental injuries

Classification systems for traumatic dental injuries provide essential frameworks for diagnosis, treatment planning, and prognosis assessment. Three primary classification systems dominate the field: Andreasen's classification, the World Health Organization (WHO) classification, and the International Association of Dental Traumatology (IADT) guidelines [15].

Andreasen's classification, widely regarded as the gold standard, offers the most comprehensive approach to categorizing dental trauma [16]. It systematically divides injuries into four main categories: injuries to hard dental tissues and pulp, injuries to periodontal tissues, injuries to supporting bone, and injuries to gingival or oral mucosa. This classification's strength lies in its detailed descriptions and inclusion of both primary and permanent dentition considerations, acknowledging that trauma often results in multiple concurrent injuries. The WHO classification system,

Category	Risk factor	Associated Risk Level	Prevention strategies
Physical	Increased overjet (>3 mm)	High	Orthodontic treatment
	Overjet >6 mm	Very High	Early intervention
	Insufficient lip coverage	Moderate-High	Oral function therapy
	Class II division 1 malocclusion	High	Orthodontic correction
Behavioral	Contact sports participation	Very High	Mouthguards, face protection
	Risk-taking behavior	High	Education, supervision
	Unsafe play practices	Moderate-High	Safety guidelines
Environmental	Unsafe playground equipment	High	Regular maintenance, padding
	Urban environment hazards	Moderate	Environmental modification
	Traffic-related risks	High	Traffic safety measures

Table 1.
Major risk factors for traumatic dental injuries.

integrated into the International Classification of Diseases (ICD), provides a more streamlined approach focused on international standardization. It categorizes injuries into three primary groups: fractures, luxation, displacement of teeth, and other injuries, including soft tissues [15]. This system's simplicity makes it particularly valuable for administrative purposes, insurance documentation, and epidemiological research.

The IADT guidelines represent a modern synthesis, combining elements of Andreasen's and WHO classifications while emphasizing practical clinical applications. These guidelines are distinctive in their focus on evidence-based treatment protocols and specific considerations for both primary and permanent dentition [17]. They provide detailed recommendations for emergency management, treatment procedures, and follow-up protocols. Dental professionals often integrate elements from all three systems to provide optimal patient care in clinical practice. Andreasen's classification typically guides detailed clinical diagnosis, the WHO system facilitates administrative documentation, and IADT guidelines inform treatment planning and management protocols [18]. This integrated approach enables comprehensive patient assessment, standardized documentation, and effective communication among healthcare providers.

3. Diagnosis and assessment

Accurate diagnosis in dental trauma requires a methodical and comprehensive approach that integrates various diagnostic modalities. The foundation of effective trauma management lies in the clinician's ability to systematically evaluate both obvious and subtle signs of injury while considering the complex interplay between hard and soft tissues. The continued evolution of diagnostic technologies promises even greater capabilities in trauma assessment and treatment planning. Emerging technologies such as photoacoustic imaging, optical coherence tomography, and advanced molecular imaging techniques are promising in providing even more detailed information about tissue status and healing potential [19]. Integrating various diagnostic modalities through artificial intelligence platforms will likely lead to increasingly sophisticated decision support systems. These systems will be capable of processing complex data from multiple sources to provide comprehensive diagnostic assessments and evidence-based treatment recommendations [20]. The development of augmented reality applications for surgical planning and guidance represents another frontier in trauma management. These technologies have the potential to provide real-time guidance during complex procedures, improving precision and reducing the risk of complications. The trend toward miniaturization and increased portability of diagnostic devices will likely continue, making advanced diagnostic capabilities more accessible in emergencies and remote settings. This development, coupled with teledentistry applications, can potentially improve access to specialist consultation and expertise in trauma management. As these technologies continue to evolve, the challenge will be to integrate them effectively into clinical practice while maintaining cost-effectiveness and practical utility [21]. The future of dental trauma diagnostics lies in the thoughtful application of these advanced tools to improve patient care and treatment outcomes, guided by sound clinical judgment and evidence-based principles. Diagnosing dental trauma effectively is the cornerstone of treatment and predicting long-term outcomes. A systematic approach incorporating various diagnostic tools and techniques is essential to evaluate the full extent of the injury. Here is a breakdown of key diagnostic approaches in dental trauma [22].

3.1 Clinical examination protocol

The initial clinical examination begins with a detailed trauma history, encompassing the mechanism of injury, time elapsed since the incident, and presenting symptoms. This information provides crucial context for understanding the potential extent and severity of the injury. The temporal relationship between trauma occurrence and clinical presentation is particularly significant in determining treatment urgency and predicting potential complications [23]. The extraoral examination evaluates facial symmetry, soft tissue injuries, and temporomandibular joint function. This assessment must be thorough yet gentle, considering the patient's comfort and potential underlying injuries. The intraoral examination focuses on both the obvious signs of trauma and subtle indicators that might suggest more serious structural damage [24]. The systematic evaluation of tooth mobility, displacement patterns, and occlusal relationships provides valuable diagnostic information.

3.2 Advanced imaging techniques

Modern radiographic examination in dental trauma has evolved to include multiple imaging modalities, each offering unique diagnostic advantages. Conventional periapical radiographs remain fundamental for initial assessment, while advanced three-dimensional imaging through Cone beam computed tomography (CBCT) provides unprecedented detail in complex cases [25]. The selection of appropriate imaging techniques must balance diagnostic necessity with radiation exposure considerations, particularly in pediatric cases.

3.2.1 Digital imaging technologies

In the rapidly evolving landscape of dental traumatology, digital imaging technologies have revolutionized the diagnostic process, providing unprecedented accuracy and detail in trauma assessment. These technological advances have transformed how dental professionals evaluate, plan, and monitor traumatic dental injuries, leading to more predictable and successful treatment outcomes [26].

3.2.2 Digital radiography

Digital radiography has undergone significant advancement, offering improved image quality, reduced radiation exposure, and enhanced diagnostic capabilities compared to conventional film-based systems. Modern digital sensors provide superior contrast resolution and dynamic range, enabling better visualization of subtle injury patterns and early detection of post-traumatic complications [4]. Advanced image processing algorithms have revolutionized digital radiography, allowing for real-time enhancement of radiographic images. Features such as contrast adjustment, edge enhancement, and noise reduction have improved the visibility of critical structures and subtle pathological changes. These capabilities are precious in detecting hairline fractures, subtle periodontal ligament (PDL) widening, and early signs of root resorption. Integrating artificial intelligence with digital radiography has led to automated image analysis tools that can assist in identifying and characterizing traumatic injuries. These systems can highlight potential areas of concern, measure root lengths and angles, and track changes over time with remarkable precision. Digital subtraction radiography, another significant advance, enables precise comparison of sequential images, facilitating the early detection of post-traumatic changes and monitoring of healing patterns [27]. The advent of wireless sensors and portable X-ray devices has improved the efficiency of emergency trauma assessment, allowing for immediate imaging even in challenging clinical situations. These technological advances have facilitated better documentation and communication between healthcare providers, enabling rapid consultation and coordinated treatment planning.

3.2.3 Cone beam computed tomography (CBCT) applications

Cone beam computed tomography has emerged as an indispensable tool in dental trauma diagnosis, offering three-dimensional visualization of dental structures with exceptional detail and precision. The technology's ability to provide high-resolution cross-sectional images has particularly enhanced assessing complex traumatic injuries. CBCT imaging offers superior visualization of root fractures, especially in cases where conventional radiography may be inconclusive due to overlapping structures or oblique fracture patterns [28]. In dental trauma, CBCT's applications extend beyond essential diagnosis. The technology enables precise evaluation of root fracture location and orientation, assessment of displacement patterns in luxation injuries, and detailed analysis of alveolar bone fractures. The three-dimensional nature of CBCT imaging allows practitioners to visualize the spatial relationship between injured teeth and adjacent anatomical structures, which is crucial for planning surgical interventions and avoiding complications [29]. CBCT has proven particularly valuable in cases involving multiple tooth injuries, where understanding the complex interplay of various trauma patterns is essential for appropriate treatment planning. The technology's ability to provide volumetric measurements has also enhanced the assessment of post-traumatic bone defects and planning for regenerative procedures. Advanced CBCT software applications now offer features such as virtual treatment simulation, enabling clinicians to predict treatment outcomes and optimize intervention strategies [30]. Recent developments in CBCT technology have focused on reducing radiation exposure while maintaining image quality. Modern systems incorporate dose optimization protocols and region-specific scanning options, addressing concerns about radiation exposure, particularly in pediatric patients. These advances have made CBCT an increasingly practical tool for initial assessment and follow-up imaging in dental trauma cases.

3.2.4 3D imaging for treatment planning

Three-dimensional imaging technology has transformed treatment planning in dental trauma cases, offering unprecedented visualization capabilities and enabling virtual treatment simulation. Advanced 3D imaging systems integrate data from multiple sources, including CBCT, surface scanning, and photographic imaging, to create comprehensive digital representations of the traumatized dentition and surrounding structures. Digital smile design principles have been adapted for trauma cases, allowing clinicians to plan esthetic rehabilitation more precisely [26]. These systems enable virtual mock-ups of proposed treatments, facilitating communication with patients and other healthcare providers. Simulating different treatment approaches and visualizing potential outcomes has proven particularly valuable in complex cases involving multiple injured teeth. Integrating 3D printing technology with treatment planning systems has enabled the fabrication of surgical guides, custom splints, and provisional restorations with exceptional accuracy. These applications have improved surgical interventions' precision and enhanced treatment outcomes' predictability. Modern 3D imaging systems also incorporate motion tracking capabilities, enabling dynamic assessment of occlusal relationships and functional movements [31]. This information is precious in cases involving displacement injuries, where understanding the impact on functional relationships is crucial for treatment planning.

3.3 Novel assessment tools

Pulp Vitality Assessment: Contemporary pulp vitality testing incorporates both traditional and advanced methods. While conventional thermal and electric pulp testing provides valuable information, newer technologies such as laser Doppler flowmetry offer a more objective assessment of pulpal blood flow [32]. The interpretation of these tests must consider the potential for false responses in recently traumatized teeth and the limitations of each testing method.

3.3.1 Pulp vitality testing innovations

The field of pulp vitality assessment has witnessed significant advancement with the introduction of novel testing methods that offer greater accuracy and reliability than traditional approaches [33]. Modern pulse oximetry devices, specifically designed for dental applications, can now provide real-time measurement of pulpal blood flow, offering a truly objective assessment of pulp vitality rather than merely testing nerve response.

3.3.2 Biomarkers for pulp and periodontal healing

Identifying and utilizing biological markers for assessing pulpal and periodontal healing represents a significant advance in trauma diagnostics. Modern molecular biology techniques have enabled the detection of specific proteins, enzymes, and inflammatory mediators that can indicate the extent of tissue damage and predict healing potential. Dentinal fluid analysis has emerged as a promising diagnostic tool, with researchers identifying specific proteins and molecules that correlate with pulpal inflammation and repair processes [34]. These biomarkers can be detected in minimally invasive samples, providing valuable information about pulpal health and the likelihood of successful conservative management. In the periodontal context, advanced diagnostic tests can now detect specific inflammatory mediators in gingival crevicular fluid, providing insights into the healing status of traumatized periodontal tissues. These molecular markers can help predict outcomes in cases of luxation injuries and guide decisions regarding the timing and nature of interventions. The development of chairside testing kits for various biomarkers has made these advanced diagnostic capabilities more accessible in clinical practice [35]. These rapid diagnostic tools can provide immediate information about tissue status, enabling more timely and appropriate therapeutic interventions.

3.3.3 Laser Doppler flowmetry (LDF)

LDF has emerged as a sophisticated tool for evaluating pulpal blood flow, particularly valuable in cases of traumatic injury where conventional sensitivity tests may be unreliable. This non-invasive technology measures blood flow by detecting Doppler-shifted wavelengths of reflected laser light, providing quantitative data about pulpal circulation [36]. The technology has proven particularly useful in monitoring recovery in traumatized teeth and predicting long-term pulpal health outcomes. Recent innovations include the development of ultrasound Doppler devices specifically designed for dental applications. These instruments offer improved depth penetration and can provide detailed information about blood flow patterns within the dental pulp [37]. Integrating these technologies with digital documentation systems allows for objective tracking of pulpal recovery over time, facilitating evidence-based decision-making regarding endodontic intervention.

3.4 AI-assisted diagnosis and treatment planning

Artificial Intelligence has emerged as a transformative force in dental trauma diagnosis and treatment planning. Machine learning algorithms, trained on vast databases of trauma cases, can now assist clinicians in injury classification, prognosis assessment, and treatment selection. These AI systems analyze complex patterns in imaging data, patient history, and clinical findings to provide evidence-based recommendations for treatment approaches. AI-powered diagnostic tools have demonstrated remarkable accuracy in detecting subtle radiographic signs of trauma, often identifying features that might be overlooked in conventional analysis [38]. These systems can automatically segment anatomical structures, measure displacement angles in luxation injuries, and quantify bone loss in traumatic injuries, providing objective data for treatment planning. Deep learning algorithms have been developed to predict treatment outcomes based on initial presentation and proposed interventions. These predictive models consider multiple variables, including patient age, injury type, time elapsed since injury, and treatment modality, to estimate the likelihood of success for different treatment approaches. This capability has proven particularly valuable in complex cases with multiple treatment options. Integrating AI with digital patient records has enabled the development of intelligent treatment planning systems that can suggest evidence-based protocols based on current best practices and patient-specific factors [39]. These systems can also alert clinicians to potential complications and recommend appropriate preventive measures or modifications to treatment plans.

3.5 Documentation and monitoring

Comprehensive documentation through clinical photography and detailed charting is essential for immediate treatment planning, healing progression, and managing potential complications. Digital photography has revolutionized trauma management, enabling precise documentation and communication between healthcare providers [40]. The diagnostic approach must be tailored to patient-specific factors, including age, developmental stage, and medical history. Pediatric cases require particular attention to the potential impact on developing permanent dentition, while adult cases may need consideration of existing restorative work and periodontal status. The availability of diagnostic resources and injury severity guide the selection of appropriate diagnostic tools and techniques [41].

4. Emergency management protocols in dental trauma

Dental trauma screening protocols have been refined to incorporate comprehensive assessment algorithms that guide clinicians through systematic evaluation of dental injuries. These protocols begin with a rapid assessment of vital signs and neurological status, which is critical in cases involving head trauma. The contemporary approach emphasizes the "ABCDE" methodology (Airway, Breathing, Circulation, Disability, Exposure) before focusing on specific dental injuries. Current screening protocols incorporate standardized documentation systems that capture essential information about the injury mechanism, timing, and circumstances. Digital documentation platforms now enable real-time recording of clinical findings, including standardized trauma scores and risk assessments. These systems often include integrated clinical decision support tools that help guide the assessment process and identify potential complications [42]. Modern protocols emphasize the importance of extra- and intraoral photography as part of initial documentation. Standardized photographic protocols ensure comprehensive documentation of visible injuries, which is crucial for treatment planning, medical purposes, and monitoring healing progress. Advanced imaging protocols consider radiation exposure guidelines while ensuring adequate diagnostic information is obtained. The integration of systematic head and neck examination has become standard in dental trauma screening, recognizing the frequent association between dental injuries and other maxillofacial trauma [43]. Contemporary protocols include specific guidelines for identifying concurrent injuries that may require immediate medical intervention or influence dental treatment planning.

4.1 Initial assessment and triage

The management of traumatic dental injuries in the emergency setting has evolved significantly with the implementation of standardized protocols and advanced technologies. Contemporary emergency management emphasizes rapid, systematic assessment and evidence-based interventions to optimize treatment outcomes [44]. The initial moments following dental trauma are crucial, and modern protocols have been developed to ensure efficient and effective emergency care delivery (**Figure 1**).

4.2 Emergency management workflow

The Emergency Management Workflow for Dental Trauma (**Figure 1**) provides a systematic approach to triaging and managing dental trauma cases. The workflow begins with the initial patient contact, leading to a critical emergency assessment phase where the severity and nature of the trauma are evaluated. From this assessment, the case is directed into one of three primary pathways based on urgency and type of injury.

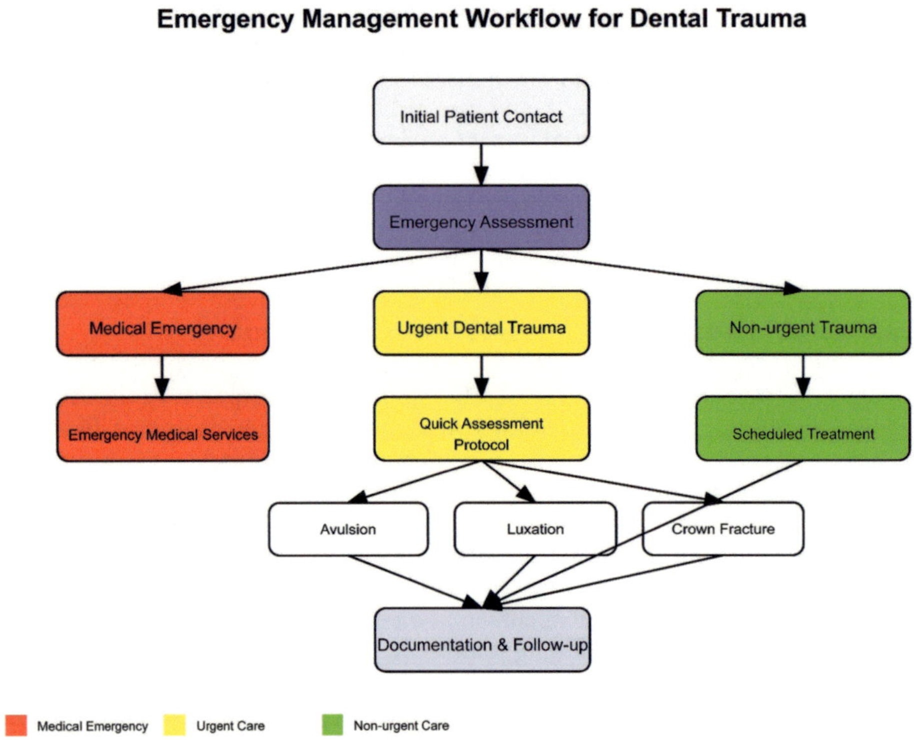

Figure 1.
Dental trauma emergency workflow chart.

The medical emergency pathway (red) addresses life-threatening conditions that require immediate medical intervention, such as severe head trauma or compromised airway. The urgent dental trauma pathway (yellow) manages immediate dental emergencies through three sub-protocols: avulsion cases requiring immediate tooth replantation, luxation injuries needing repositioning, and crown fractures requiring immediate pain management and pulp protection. The non-urgent pathway (green) handles less time-sensitive cases that can be managed through scheduled treatment.

All pathways ultimately converge at the documentation and follow-up stage, ensuring comprehensive record-keeping and appropriate monitoring of treatment outcomes. The workflow emphasizes the importance of proper case categorization and protocol adherence while maintaining flexibility to address individual patient needs. Directional arrows indicate the flow of decision-making and patient management, with potential feedback loops where reassessment may be necessary. This workflow serves as a quick reference guide for dental professionals, ensuring systematic and evidence-based management of dental trauma cases while prioritizing patient safety and optimal treatment outcomes. The color-coding system allows for rapid identification of appropriate pathways during emergency situations, facilitating efficient and effective patient care.

4.3 Emergency prioritization guidelines

Emergency prioritization systems in dental trauma have evolved to incorporate evidence-based triage protocols that help clinicians determine the urgency of various injury types. These systems typically classify injuries into immediate, urgent, and non-urgent categories, with specific time-sensitive interventions identified for each category. Contemporary guidelines emphasize the importance of early recognition of time-critical injuries, particularly avulsion, severe luxation, and alveolar fractures [45]. Digital triage systems now incorporate algorithms that help clinicians quickly identify high-priority cases and determine appropriate intervention timing. These systems often include automatic alerting mechanisms for cases requiring immediate specialist consultation. The development of standardized emergency care pathways has improved the efficiency of trauma management. These pathways provide clear guidance on the sequence of interventions, considering factors such as multiple injury patterns, patient age, and medical status. Modern protocols also include specific primary versus permanent dentition considerations, recognizing the different management approaches required for each [46]. Risk stratification has become an integral component of emergency prioritization, with protocols incorporating assessment of factors that may influence treatment outcomes. These include evaluating medical complications, assessing cooperation potential (particularly in pediatric cases), and considering resource availability.

4.4 Modern storage media for avulsed teeth

The science of tooth storage media has advanced significantly, with new solutions designed to maintain PDL cell viability and improve replantation outcomes. Contemporary storage media incorporate balanced osmolality, pH, and nutritional factors optimized for PDL cell survival. Commercial products now include specific formulations for different storage durations and transport conditions [47]. Advanced storage solutions often contain growth factors and cell-protective compounds that help maintain PDL cell viability during extraoral periods. Research has led to the development of storage media with enhanced antimicrobial properties while maintaining biocompatibility [48]. These solutions often include indicators that change color based on storage duration or media effectiveness. The development of ready-to-use tooth storage kits has improved the emergency management of avulsion cases. These kits typically include storage solutions, handling instructions, and documentation materials. Some advanced kits incorporate temperature-stable formulations and extended shelf-life capabilities, making them practical for inclusion in first-aid kits and emergency facilities [49].

4.5 Immediate stabilization techniques

Contemporary stabilization approaches emphasize minimally invasive techniques that promote optimal healing while maintaining physiologic tooth mobility. Modern splinting materials include fiber-reinforced composites and advanced resin materials that provide adequate stabilization and are easy to apply and remove [50]. These materials often incorporate antibacterial properties and release therapeutic agents to support healing. Digital technology has enabled the development of custom-fabricated splints using CAD/CAM systems, allowing for precise fit and optimal force distribution. These systems can rapidly produce splints, even in emergencies, improving the accuracy and efficiency of stabilization procedures [51]. Some advanced systems incorporate sensors that monitor splinting forces and tooth mobility during healing. Integrating bioactive materials in stabilization techniques represents a significant advance in trauma management. These materials can promote healing while providing mechanical support [52]. Modern protocols emphasize the importance of appropriate splinting duration based on injury type and healing progress, with some systems incorporating indicators for optimal splint removal timing.

4.6 Pain management protocols

Contemporary pain management in dental trauma has evolved to incorporate multi-modal approaches that address both immediate and ongoing pain control needs. Modern protocols emphasize using evidence-based analgesic regimens tailored to injury severity and patient factors. Advanced local anesthetic techniques, including computer-controlled delivery systems and long-acting formulations, have improved acute pain management in trauma cases [53]. The development of targeted pain control strategies has led to more effective management of different pain types associated with dental trauma. These protocols often incorporate pharmacological and non-pharmacological approaches, including advanced delivery systems for local drug administration. Some protocols now include specific considerations for managing pain in different age groups and medical conditions [54]. Digital pain assessment tools have improved the effectiveness of pain control monitoring and documentation. These systems often incorporate real-time pain scoring and medication tracking, enabling more precise adjustment of pain management strategies [55]. Modern protocols also emphasize the importance of preventing chronic pain development through appropriate early intervention.

4.7 Remote consultation technologies

The integration of teledentistry and remote consultation platforms has revolutionized emergency dental trauma management. These technologies enable rapid access to specialist expertise, particularly valuable in settings where immediate specialist care is unavailable [56]. Modern platforms incorporate secure video consultation capabilities, allowing real-time assessment and guidance from trauma specialists. Digital imaging sharing systems enable rapid transmission of radiographs and clinical photographs to consulting specialists, facilitating immediate expert input on complex cases. These systems often include real-time annotation and discussion features, improving communication between primary care providers and specialists. Mobile applications designed specifically for dental trauma have emerged as valuable tools for clinicians and patients [57]. These apps often include emergency management guidelines, documentation tools, and direct communication channels with specialist providers. Some applications incorporate artificial intelligence algorithms that can assist in initial injury assessment and triage decisions.

5. Treatment strategies

5.1 Regenerative endodontic procedures

The field of regenerative endodontics has revolutionized the treatment approach for traumatized teeth, particularly in cases involving immature permanent teeth with incomplete root development. These innovative procedures aim to restore tooth vitality and promote continued root development, offering alternatives to traditional endodontic treatments.

5.2 Stem cell therapy applications

Stem cell therapy has emerged as a ground-breaking approach in dental trauma management, offering unprecedented tissue regeneration and repair possibilities. Dental pulp stem cells (DPSCs) stem cells from human exfoliated deciduous teeth (SHED) and periodontal ligament stem cells (PDLSCs) have shown remarkable potential in regenerating damaged dental tissues [58]. These multipotent cells can differentiate into various cell types, including odontoblasts, cementoblasts, and PDL fibroblasts. Recent advances in stem cell isolation and cultivation techniques have made clinical applications more feasible. Advanced protocols now exist for harvesting, expanding, and storing dental stem cells for therapeutic use. Developing novel scaffolds and delivery systems has improved the integration and survival of transplanted stem cells [59]. Research has demonstrated successful outcomes in regenerating pulp-dentin complex, periodontal tissues, and even entire tooth structures. Current applications include autologous stem cell transplantation for pulp regeneration in necrotic immature teeth, periodontal regeneration following traumatic injuries, and bone regeneration in cases of severe alveolar damage. Integrating growth factors and bioactive molecules with stem cell therapy has enhanced treatment outcomes, promoting more predictable tissue regeneration [60].

5.3 Pulp revascularization techniques

Modern pulp revascularization protocols have evolved significantly, incorporating evidence-based approaches to promote pulp tissue regeneration. Contemporary techniques utilize controlled bleeding from the periapical tissues to create a scaffold rich in growth factors and stem cells [61]. Advanced irrigation protocols, including using modified concentrations of antimicrobial solutions, help maintain stem cell viability while ensuring adequate disinfection. Introducing plasma-rich proteins and other biological modifiers has enhanced the success rates of revascularization procedures [62]. These techniques often incorporate carefully selected bioactive materials to create an optimal environment for tissue regeneration. Modern protocols emphasize the importance of coronal seal integrity, utilizing advanced materials that promote tissue ingrowth while preventing bacterial contamination. Follow-up protocols now include advanced imaging techniques to monitor the progress of root development and tissue regeneration [63]. Digital volumetric analysis allows for precise measurement of continued root development and assessment of tissue mineralization patterns.

5.4 Bioactive materials in regeneration

The development of bioactive materials has transformed regenerative endodontic procedures. Modern calcium silicate-based materials, bioceramics, and glass ionomers incorporate properties that actively promote tissue healing and regeneration [64]. These materials often release therapeutic ions that stimulate cellular differentiation and tissue mineralization. Advanced hydrogel scaffolds and injectable materials provide a controlled release of growth factors and antimicrobial agents. Smart materials that respond to environmental changes can modify their properties to optimize healing conditions. Integrating nanoparticles and bioactive molecules has enhanced the therapeutic potential of these materials [65].

5.5 Advanced splinting techniques

5.5.1 Innovative materials in dental splinting

The introduction of innovative materials has revolutionized dental splinting techniques. These materials can respond to environmental changes, providing dynamic support during healing. Shape memory alloys and polymers offer controlled force application and can adjust their properties based on healing progression [66]. Contemporary splinting materials often incorporate monitoring capabilities, allowing clinicians to track healing progress and adjust treatment accordingly. Some advanced materials change color or properties to indicate optimal removal timing or excessive force application. Developing bioactive splinting materials that release therapeutic agents has improved healing outcomes [67].

5.5.2 Fiber-reinforced composites

Modern fiber-reinforced composites (FRCs) offer superior mechanical properties while maintaining excellent esthetics and ease of application. These materials provide optimal force distribution and can be customized for specific clinical situations. Advanced fiber designs and resin formulations have improved handling characteristics and bonding properties [68]. Recent developments include antibacterial fibers and materials with enhanced biocompatibility. Some FRCs now incorporate remineralizing agents and growth factors to promote tissue healing [69]. Computer-optimized fiber orientations provide improved stress distribution and mechanical properties.

5.5.3 Computer-aided splint design

Digital technology has transformed splint design and fabrication. CAD/CAM systems enable the creation of precisely fitted splints that optimize force distribution and patient comfort. Virtual planning allows for the simulation of different designs and the prediction of biomechanical effects. 3D printing technology has made rapid fabrication of custom splints possible, even in emergencies [70]. Advanced software can analyze occlusal forces and tooth mobility to optimize splint design. Integration with patient monitoring systems allows for remote adjustment of treatment parameters.

5.6 Surgical interventions

5.6.1 Microsurgical approaches

Modern microsurgical techniques have significantly improved the precision and predictability of dental trauma surgery. Operating microscopes and enhanced magnification systems provide superior visualization of fine anatomical structures [71]. Advanced microsurgical instruments enable minimally invasive approaches with reduced tissue trauma. The integration of digital imaging and navigation systems has enhanced surgical accuracy. Real-time monitoring capabilities allow for precise control of surgical procedures. Advanced wound closure techniques and materials have improved healing outcomes [72].

5.6.2 Guided tissue regeneration

Contemporary guided tissue regeneration (GTR) techniques incorporate advanced barrier membranes and biomaterials. Novel membrane designs provide optimal space maintenance while allowing for selective cell population growth. Smart membranes can respond to local tissue conditions and release therapeutic agents [73]. The development of customized scaffolds using 3D printing technology has improved the precision of tissue regeneration. Integration of growth factors and bioactive molecules enhances regenerative outcomes. Advanced imaging techniques enable precise monitoring of tissue regeneration progress [74].

5.6.3 Autotransplantation

Modern autotransplantation procedures benefit from improved surgical planning and execution techniques. Digital planning software enables precise donor tooth selection and recipient site preparation. 3D-printed surgical guides improve the accuracy of transplantation procedures. Advanced preservation solutions and techniques have improved the success rates of autotransplantation. The development of bioactive materials for root surface treatment enhances periodontal healing. Integration with regenerative techniques provides better outcomes in complex cases [75].

6. Trauma prevention and risk management

6.1 Recognition and pattern analysis in risk factor assessment

The comprehensive understanding and systematic analysis of risk factors in traumatic dental injuries (TDI) constitute a fundamental cornerstone in developing effective prevention and management strategies. Recognizing these patterns enables healthcare providers to implement evidence-based approaches that address immediate and long-term prevention needs. Through sophisticated epidemiological analysis and clinical observation, practitioners can develop targeted interventions considering the multifaceted nature of dental trauma risk factors [76]. In the contemporary healthcare landscape, the identification of risk patterns has evolved from simple observational methods to complex analytical approaches incorporating artificial intelligence and big data analysis. This evolution has enhanced our ability to predict and prevent traumatic dental injuries across diverse populations. Integrating multiple data sources, including clinical records, demographic information, and environmental factors, allows for more precise risk stratification and personalized prevention strategies [7].

6.2 Evidence-based prevention strategies

The systematic management of risk factors in dental trauma prevention represents a complex interplay of clinical expertise, public health principles, and evidence-based practice. Through carefully integrating these elements, healthcare providers can significantly improve prevention effectiveness and treatment outcomes. Developing targeted interventions based on systematic risk analysis has led to more efficient and effective prevention strategies [77]. This comprehensive approach to understanding and managing risk factors continues to evolve with advancing technology and improving understanding of trauma mechanisms. Integrating digital health technologies, artificial intelligence, and precision medicine principles promises to enhance further our ability to prevent and manage traumatic dental injuries effectively [44]. Through this sophisticated approach to risk factor analysis and management, dental traumatology continues to advance, providing increasingly effective strategies for preventing and managing dental injuries across diverse populations and healthcare settings.

6.3 Physical risk factor management

Managing physical risk factors in dental trauma prevention requires a sophisticated, multidisciplinary approach incorporating contemporary orthodontic principles and preventive dentistry concepts. Early orthodontic intervention, particularly in increased overjet and malocclusion cases, represents a primary prevention strategy supported by extensive clinical evidence [78]. Implementing regular dental surveillance protocols and incorporating advanced diagnostic technologies enables early identification of anatomical risk factors and timely intervention. The assessment of oral protection needs has evolved to include comprehensive biomechanical analysis and customized protective device design. Modern approaches utilize digital scanning and computer-aided design to create precisely fitted protective devices that optimize protection and comfort [79]. These advanced techniques have significantly improved the effectiveness of physical protection strategies while enhancing patient compliance.

6.4 Behavioral risk factor modification

Contemporary behavioral modification approaches in dental trauma prevention integrate psychology, sports medicine, and public health principles. Educational programs have evolved beyond simple information dissemination to incorporate interactive learning technologies and behavior change theories. These programs utilize evidence-based methodologies to achieve sustainable behavioral modifications that reduce trauma risk [1]. The development of sports safety protocols now incorporates advanced risk assessment tools and real-time monitoring systems. Behavioral modification programs utilize cognitive-behavioral techniques and motivational interviewing to achieve better compliance with safety measures. Regular risk assessment protocols incorporate standardized evaluation tools and digital monitoring systems to track behavioral changes and intervention effectiveness [80].

6.5 Environmental risk management

Environmental risk management in dental trauma prevention requires a systematic approach incorporating public health, urban planning, and safety engineering principles. Safety audit protocols have evolved to include sophisticated risk assessment tools and digital documentation systems. Infrastructure improvements are planned using evidence-based design principles that prioritize injury prevention while maintaining functionality [4]. Regular maintenance programs now incorporate predictive analytics to identify potential hazards before they lead to injuries.

Integrating digital communication systems and standardized response procedures has enhanced emergency response protocols. These advanced approaches ensure more effective environmental risk management and improved emergency response capabilities.

6.6 Management of recurrent trauma cases

The identification and management of repeated trauma cases require a sophisticated approach that considers multiple underlying factors. Contemporary management protocols incorporate comprehensive medical evaluation, psychological assessment, and environmental analysis [81]. Recognizing potential abuse situations has been enhanced by developing standardized screening protocols and improved interdisciplinary communication systems.

6.7 Implementation of comprehensive prevention strategies

Implementing prevention strategies in modern dental trauma management requires careful consideration of multiple factors affecting intervention effectiveness. Individual risk assessment protocols now incorporate advanced diagnostic tools and predictive analytics. Age-appropriate interventions are designed using evidence-based developmental principles and contemporary educational theories. To ensure intervention appropriateness, cultural and social factors are evaluated using sophisticated anthropological and sociological frameworks [82].

7. Future directions in dental trauma management

The landscape of dental trauma management is rapidly evolving, driven by unprecedented technological advances and deepening biological insights. Emergency management protocols' continued evolution incorporates several key developments that promise to transform the field.

7.1 Technological integration

Integrating artificial intelligence-driven decision support systems and augmented reality guidance for emergency procedures is revolutionizing treatment approaches. These digital innovations, combined with expanding teledentistry capabilities and remote monitoring systems, are improving access to specialized trauma care, particularly in underserved areas [44, 83]. The integration of emergency protocols with electronic health records and digital documentation systems continues to enhance the efficiency and effectiveness of trauma management.

7.2 Advanced materials and treatments

The development of new bioactive materials and smart delivery systems for medications promises to improve treatment outcomes. The field is witnessing a paradigm shift through the integration of advanced biomaterials, gene therapy, and personalized medicine approaches. These innovations are expanding the possibilities for tissue regeneration and functional restoration.

7.3 Evidence-based practice and research

Implementing innovative treatment strategies demands rigorous scientific validation through comprehensive research protocols. Contemporary investigations focus on:

- Evaluating long-term outcomes
- Comparing treatment effectiveness
- Analyzing cost-benefit ratios of advanced therapeutic modalities
- Establishing robust systems for monitoring and evaluating treatment outcomes

This systematic approach to evidence generation ensures that new treatment protocols are clinically effective, economically viable, and practically implementable across diverse healthcare settings.

7.4 Professional development and implementation

The complexity of modern trauma management necessitates a sophisticated understanding of both traditional principles and emerging technologies. Success in this evolving landscape depends on:

- Appropriate case selection
- Advanced professional training
- Strategic investment in technology and infrastructure
- Continuous professional education and skill development
- Development of comprehensive clinical protocols

Healthcare providers must incorporate these new modalities while ensuring patient education and compliance. The impact of these developments extends beyond immediate treatment outcomes to encompass broader considerations of healthcare delivery, professional education, and patient engagement.

As the field advances, the synthesis of biological understanding and technological innovation creates unprecedented opportunities for improving treatment outcomes. However, these advances must be balanced with practical considerations of cost-effectiveness and accessibility to ensure the widespread implementation of optimal care protocols. The future of dental trauma management lies in the thoughtful application of these advanced techniques, always guided by evidence-based principles and focused on delivering predictable, cost-effective, and patient-centered care.

Dental traumatology stands at the threshold of transformative change, promising enhanced therapeutic possibilities while maintaining its fundamental commitment to patient care excellence. This systematic approach, combining scientific rigor with clinical pragmatism, ensures that innovations in dental trauma treatment translate effectively into improved patient outcomes.

DOI: http://dx.doi.org/10.5772/intechopen.1009439

Author details

Anil Sukumaran[1,2] and Betsy Joseph[3,4*]

1 Oral Health Institute, Hamad Medical Corporation, Doha, Qatar

2 College of Dental Medicine, Qatar University, Doha, Qatar

3 Department of Periodontology, Saveetha Dental College and Hospitals, Saveetha Institute of Medical and Technical Sciences, Saveetha University, Chennai, India

4 Department of Oral and Maxillofacial Diseases, Helsinki University and University Hospital, Helsinki, Finland

*Address all correspondence to: jobets121@gmail.com

References

[1] Brandini DA, de Souza C, Cantao AB, Levin L. Public health policies in dental traumatology: A call for action! Dental Traumatology. 2024;**40**(6):612-617

[2] Petti S, Glendor U, Andersson L. World traumatic dental injury prevalence and incidence, a meta-analysis—One billion living people have had traumatic dental injuries. Dental Traumatology. 2018;**34**(2):71-86

[3] Tysiac-Mista M, Tanasiewicz M, Amini S, Najary S, Baghani MT, Eftekhar Ashtiani R, et al. Traumatic dental injuries' prevalence across diverse healthcare settings: A systematic review and meta-analysis. Archives of Academic Emergency Medicine. 2025;**13**(1):e11

[4] Khan MK, Jindal MK. Assessment of the environmental risk factors associated with traumatic dental injuries among WHO index-aged children and adolescents. Journal of Education Health Promotion. 2023;**12**:396

[5] Glendor U. Epidemiology of traumatic dental injuries–A 12 year review of the literature. Dental Traumatology. 2008;**24**(6):603-611

[6] Abbott P. Traumatic dental injuries are now the 5th most prevalent disease/injury in the world-but they are being neglected!! Dental Traumatology. 2018;**34**(6):383

[7] Nagarajappa R, Ramesh G, Uthappa R, Kannan SPK, Shaikh S. Risk factors and patterns of traumatic dental injuries among Indian adolescents. Journal of Dental Sciences. 2020;**15**(1):96-103

[8] Abdel Malak C, Chakar C, Romanos A, Rachidi S. Prevalence and etiological factors of dental trauma among 12- and 15-year-old schoolchildren of Lebanon: A National Study. Scientific World Journal. 2021;**2021**:5587431

[9] Aldrigui JM, Jabbar NS, Bonecker M, Braga MM, Wanderley MT. Trends and associated factors in prevalence of dental trauma in Latin America and Caribbean: A systematic review and meta-analysis. Community Dentistry and Oral Epidemiology. 2014;**42**(1):30-42

[10] Lembacher S, Schneider S, Lettner S, Bekes K. Prevalence and patterns of traumatic dental injuries in the permanent dentition: A three-year retrospective overview study at the university dental clinic of Vienna. International Journal of Environmental Research and Public Health. 2022;**19**(23):1-10

[11] Lam R. Epidemiology and outcomes of traumatic dental injuries: A review of the literature. Australian Dental Journal. 2016;**61**(Suppl. 1(S1)):4-20

[12] Răzvan GC, Costan VV, Boisteanu O, Armencia A, Ciofu M, Balcos C, et al. Traumatic dental injuries among adolescents and young adults in Iași, Romania: Legal and medical perspectives. Dentistry Journal. 2024;**12**(9):282

[13] Dolic O, Obradovic M, Kojic Z, Knezevic N, Trtic N, Veselinovic V, et al. Traumatic dental injuries in children and adolescents from a major dental Clinic in Bosnia and Herzegovina: A 5-year retrospective study. Medicina. 2024;**60**(11):1843

[14] Glendor U. Aetiology and risk factors related to traumatic dental injuries–A review of the literature. Dental Traumatology. 2009;**25**(1):19-31

[15] Petti S, Andreasen JO, Glendor U, Andersson L. NA0D - The new traumatic dental injury classification of the World Health Organization. Dental Traumatology. 2022;**38**(3):170-174

[16] Abbott PV. The World Health Organization recognizes the Andreasen classification of traumatic dental injuries. Dental Traumatology. 2022;**38**(3):169

[17] Day PF, Flores MT, O'Connell AC, Abbott PV, Tsilingaridis G, Fouad AF, et al. International Association of Dental Traumatology guidelines for the management of traumatic dental injuries: 3. Injuries in the primary dentition. Dental Traumatology. 2020;**36**(4):343-359

[18] Andreasen FM, Kahler B. Diagnosis of acute dental trauma: The importance of standardized documentation: A review. Dental Traumatology. 2015;**31**(5):340-349

[19] Bakland LK, Andreasen JO. Dental traumatology: Essential diagnosis and treatment planning. Endodontic Topics. 2004;**7**(1):14-34

[20] Musleh D, Almossaeed H, Balhareth F, Alqahtani G, Alobaidan N, Altalag J, et al. Advancing dental diagnostics: A review of artificial intelligence applications and challenges in dentistry. Big Data and Cognitive Computing. 2024;**8**(6):66

[21] Dubron K, Verbist M, Jacobs R, Olszewski R, Shaheen E, Willaert R. Augmented and virtual reality for preoperative trauma planning, focusing on orbital reconstructions: A systematic review. Journal of Clinical Medicine. 2023;**12**(16):5203

[22] Patel S, Puri T, Mannocci F, Navai A. Diagnosis and management of traumatic dental injuries using intraoral radiography and cone-beam computed tomography: An In vivo investigation. Journal of Endodontia. 2021;**47**(6):914-923

[23] Lin S, Pilosof N, Karawani M, Wigler R, Kaufman AY, Teich ST. Occurrence and timing of complications following traumatic dental injuries: A retrospective study in a dental trauma department. Journal of Clinical and Experimental Dentistry. 2016;**8**(4):e429-e436

[24] Esonu O, Sardesai MG. Initial assessment of the facial trauma patient. Seminars in Plastic Surgery. 2021;**35**(4):225-228

[25] Cohenca N, Silberman A. Contemporary imaging for the diagnosis and treatment of traumatic dental injuries: A review. Dental Traumatology. 2017;**33**(5):321-328

[26] Van Gorp G, Lambrechts M, Jacobs R, Declerck D. Does clinical experience with dental traumatology impact 2D and 3D radiodiagnostic performance in paediatric dentists? An exploratory study. BMC Oral Health. 2022;**22**(1):245

[27] Lima TF, Gamba TO, Zaia AA, Soares AJ. Evaluation of cone beam computed tomography and periapical radiography in the diagnosis of root resorption. Australian Dental Journal. 2016;**61**(4):425-431

[28] Jacobs R, Quirynen M. Dental cone beam computed tomography: Justification for use in planning oral implant placement. Periodontology 2000. 2014;**66**(1):203-213

[29] Krastl G, Weiger R, Filippi A, Van Waes H, Ebeleseder K, Ree M, et al. Endodontic management of traumatized permanent teeth: A comprehensive

review. International Endodontic Journal. 2021;**54**(8):1221-1245

[30] Rashid A, Feinberg L, Fan K. The application of cone beam computed tomography (CBCT) on the diagnosis and management of maxillofacial trauma. Diagnostics (Basel). 2024;**14**(4):373

[31] Schierz O, Hirsch C, Krey KF, Ganss C, Kammerer PW, Schlenz MA. Digital dentistry and its impact on oral health-related quality of life. The Journal of Evidence-Based Dental Practice. 2024;**24**(1S):101946

[32] Afkhami F, Wright PP, Chien PY, Xu C, Walsh LJ, Peters OA. Exploring approaches to pulp vitality assessment: A scoping review of nontraditional methods. International Endodontic Journal. 2024;**57**(8):1065-1098

[33] Patro S, Meto A, Mohanty A, Chopra V, Miglani S, Das A, et al. Diagnostic accuracy of pulp vitality tests and pulp sensibility tests for assessing pulpal health in permanent teeth: A systematic review and meta-analysis. International Journal of Environmental Research and Public Health. 2022;**19**(15):1-20

[34] Kritikou K, Imre M, Tanase M, Vinereanu A, Totan AR, Spinu T-C, et al. Biochemical mapping of the inflamed human dental pulp. Applied Sciences. 2021;**11**(21):10395

[35] Johnson RM, Tewari N, Kumar V, Rahul M, Mathur VP, Bhawal UK. Inflammatory mediators for predicting the risk of trauma-induced root resorption: A systematic review. Dental Traumatology. 2023;**39**(3):264-275

[36] Lee JY, Yanpiset K, Sigurdsson A, Vann WF Jr. Laser Doppler flowmetry for monitoring traumatized teeth. Dental Traumatology. 2001;**17**(5):231-235

[37] Ahn SY, Kim D, Park SH. Long-term prognosis of pulpal status of traumatized teeth exhibiting contradictory results between pulp sensibility test and ultrasound Doppler flowmetry: A retrospective study. Journal of Endodontia. 2018;**44**(3):395-404

[38] Karalis VD. The integration of artificial intelligence into clinical practice. Applied Biosciences. 2024;**3**(1):14-44

[39] Ozden I, Gokyar M, Ozden ME, Sazak OH. Assessment of artificial intelligence applications in responding to dental trauma. Dental Traumatology. 2024;**40**(6):722-729

[40] Tzimpoulas N, Sotiropoulou S, Tewari N. Clinical photography and documentation after traumatic dental injuries. Dental Traumatology. 2025;**41**:4-16

[41] Nemat SM, Kenny KP, Day PF. Special considerations in paediatric dental trauma. Primary Dental Journal. 2023;**12**(4):64-71

[42] Levin L, Day PF, Hicks L, O'Connell A, Fouad AF, Bourguignon C, et al. International Association of Dental Traumatology guidelines for the management of traumatic dental injuries: General introduction. Dental Traumatology. 2020;**36**(4):309-313

[43] Whyte A, Boeddinghaus R, Matias MATJ. Diagnostic imaging principles and applications in head and neck pathology. In: Farah CS, Balasubramaniam R, McCullough MJ, editors. Contemporary Oral Medicine. Cham: Springer International Publishing; 2017. pp. 1-80

[44] Zaror C, Seiffert A, Deana NF, Espinoza-Espinoza G, Atala-Acevedo C, Diaz R, et al. Emergency and sequalae management of traumatic dental

injuries: A systematic survey of clinical practice guidelines. BMC Oral Health. 2023;**23**(1):704

[45] Alnaggar D, Andersson L. Emergency management of traumatic dental injuries in 42 countries. Dental Traumatology. 2015;**31**(2):89-96

[46] Flores MT, Andersson L, Andreasen JO, Bakland LK, Malmgren B, Barnett F, et al. Guidelines for the management of traumatic dental injuries. I. Fractures and luxations of permanent teeth. Endodontic Topics. 2006;**14**(1):102-110

[47] Osmanovic A, Halilovic S, Kurtovic-Kozaric A, Hadziabdic N. Evaluation of periodontal ligament cell viability in different storage media based on human PDL cell culture experiments-a systematic review. Dental Traumatology. 2018;**34**(6):384-393

[48] Nam OH, Ro ST, Lee HW, Jeong J, Chae YK, Lee KE, et al. Evaluation of delphinidin as a storage medium for avulsed teeth. BMC Oral Health. 2023;**23**(1):21

[49] Al Sheeb M, Al Jawad FA, Nazzal H. Parents' knowledge of emergency management of avulsed permanent teeth in children and adolescents in the State of Qatar: A questionnaire cross-sectional study. European Archives of Paediatric Dentistry. 2023;**24**(5):643-650

[50] Rauch A, Mehlhorn S, Muhle M, Ziebolz D. A glass fiber-reinforced resin composite splint to stabilize and replace teeth in a periodontally compromised patient. Case Reports in Dentistry. 2020;**2020**:8886418

[51] Hinckfuss SE, Messer LB. Splinting duration and periodontal outcomes for replanted avulsed teeth: A systematic review. Dental Traumatology. 2009;**25**(2):150-157

[52] De Agustin Del Burgo JM, Blaya Haro F, D'Amato R, Juanes Mendez JA. Development of a smart splint to monitor different parameters during the treatment process. Sensors (Basel). 2020;**20**(15):4207

[53] Harvin JA, Albarado R, VTT T, Green C, Tyson JE, Pedroza C, et al. Multi-modal analgesic strategy for trauma: A pragmatic randomized clinical trial. Journal of the American College of Surgeons. 2021;**232**(3):241-251 e243

[54] Shi Y, Wu W. Multimodal non-invasive non-pharmacological therapies for chronic pain: Mechanisms and progress. BMC Medicine. 2023;**21**(1):372

[55] El-Tallawy SN, Pergolizzi JV, Vasiliu-Feltes I, Ahmed RS, LeQuang JK, El-Tallawy HN, et al. Incorporation of "artificial intelligence" for objective pain assessment: A comprehensive review. Pain and Therapy. 2024;**13**(3):293-317

[56] Sharma H, Suprabha BS, Rao A. Teledentistry and its applications in paediatric dentistry: A literature review. Pediatric Dental Journal. 2021;**31**(3):203-215

[57] Alotaibi S, Alshehri A. Teledentistry approaches for dental assessments and consultation during the COVID-19 pandemic. Smart Homecare Technology and TeleHealth. 2022;**9**(null):11-25

[58] Mattei V, Delle MS. Dental pulp stem cells (DPSCs) and tissue regeneration: Mechanisms mediated by direct, paracrine, or autocrine effects. Biomedicine. 2023;**11**(2):1-4

[59] Zhang W, Yelick PC. Tooth repair and regeneration: Potential of dental stem cells. Trends in Molecular Medicine. 2021;**27**(5):501-511

[60] Li XL, Fan W, Fan B. Dental pulp regeneration strategies: A review of

status quo and recent advances. Bioactive Materials. 2024;**38**:258-275

[61] Thalakiriyawa DS, Dissanayaka WL. Advances in regenerative dentistry approaches: An update. International Dental Journal. 2024;**74**(1):25-34

[62] Staffoli S, Plotino G, Nunez Torrijos BG, Grande NM, Bossu M, Gambarini G, et al. Regenerative endodontic procedures using contemporary endodontic materials. Materials (Basel). 2019;**12**(6):1-28

[63] Shi X, Hu X, Jiang N, Mao J. Regenerative endodontic therapy: From laboratory bench to clinical practice. Journal of Advanced Research. 2025:1-35, S2090-1232(24)00267-4

[64] Liu H, Lu J, Jiang Q, Haapasalo M, Qian J, Tay FR, et al. Biomaterial scaffolds for clinical procedures in endodontic regeneration. Bioactive Materials. 2022;**12**:257-277

[65] Choi H, Choi W-S, Jeong J-O. A review of advanced hydrogel applications for tissue engineering and drug delivery systems as biomaterials. Gels. 2024;**10**(11):693

[66] Sajjad R, Chauhdary ST, Anwar MT, Zahid A, Khosa AA, Imran M, et al. A review of 4D printing – Technologies, shape shifting, smart polymer based materials, and biomedical applications. Advanced Industrial and Engineering Polymer Research. 2024;7(1):20-36

[67] Sobczak-Zagalska H, Emerich K. Best splinting methods in case of dental injury-a literature review. The Journal of Clinical Pediatric Dentistry. 2020;**44**(2):71-78

[68] Khan AA, Zafar MS, Fareed MA, AlMufareh NA, Alshehri F, AlSunbul H, et al. Fiber-reinforced composites in dentistry - An insight into adhesion aspects of the material and the restored tooth construct. Dental Materials. 2023;**39**(2):141-151

[69] Alshabib A, Abid Althaqafi K, AlMoharib HS, Mirah M, AlFawaz YF, Algamaiah H. Dental fiber-post systems: An in-depth review of their evolution, current practice and future directions. Bioengineering. 2023;**10**(5):551

[70] Wang XT, Yang X, Guo HQ, Wang KW, Wang J, Ji AP, et al. Clinical application of CAD/CAM technology in 3D printed dental model used for removable splints fabrication in the treatment of traumatized anterior permanent teeth in children. Journal of Dentistry. 2024;**151**:105404

[71] Doppalapudi N, Burugapalli RK. Benefits of utilization of magnification in dentistry: A review. Dental Research and Oral Health. 2020;**3**(3):121-128

[72] Geo TD, Saxena P, Gupta S. Static vs. dynamic navigation for endodontic microsurgery - A comparative review. Journal of Oral Biology and Craniofacial Research. 2022;**12**(4):410-412

[73] Sasaki JI, Abe GL, Li A, Thongthai P, Tsuboi R, Kohno T, et al. Barrier membranes for tissue regeneration in dentistry. Biomaterial Investigations in Dentistry. 2021;**8**(1):54-63

[74] Selim M, Mousa HM, Abdel-Jaber GT, Barhoum A, Abdal-hay A. Innovative designs of 3D scaffolds for bone tissue regeneration: Understanding principles and addressing challenges. European Polymer Journal. 2024;**215**:113251

[75] Cross D, El-Angbawi A, McLaughlin P, Keightley A, Brocklebank L, Whitters J, et al. Developments in autotransplantation of teeth. The Surgeon. 2013;**11**(1):49-55

[76] Feldens CA, Borges TS, Vargas-Ferreira F, Kramer PF. Risk factors for traumatic dental injuries in the primary dentition: Concepts, interpretation, and evidence. Dental Traumatology. 2016;**32**(6):429-437

[77] Sigurdsson A. Evidence-based review of prevention of dental injuries. Journal of Endodontia. 2013;**39**(Suppl. 3):S88-S93

[78] Alam MK, Awawdeh M, Aljhani AS, Alotaib GS, Abutayyem H, Alswairki HJ, et al. Impact of dental trauma on orthodontic parameters - A systematic review and meta-analysis. Children (Basel). 2023;**10**(5):1-15

[79] Nasrollahzadeh N, Pioletti DP, Broome M. Design of customized mouthguards with superior protection using digital-based technologies and impact tests. Sports Medicine - Open. 2024;**10**(1):64

[80] Swann C, Rosenbaum S, Lawrence A, Vella SA, McEwan D, Ekkekakis P. Updating goal-setting theory in physical activity promotion: A critical conceptual review. Health Psychology Review. 2021;**15**(1):34-50

[81] Bourguignon C, Cohenca N, Lauridsen E, Flores MT, O'Connell AC, Day PF, et al. International Association of Dental Traumatology guidelines for the management of traumatic dental injuries: 1. Fractures and luxations. Dental Traumatology. 2020;**36**(4):314-330

[82] Bossu M, Covello F, Di Giorgio G, Zampogna S, Talarico V, De Filippo S, et al. Evaluation of the application of Italian National Guidelines for prevention and Management of Dental Injuries in developmental age. International Journal of Environmental Research and Public Health. 2020;**17**(8):1-10

[83] Nowosielska M, Baginska J, Kobus A, Kierklo A. How to educate the public about dental trauma-a scoping review. International Journal of Environmental Research and Public Health. 2022;**19**(4):1-14

Chapter 2

Vertical Root Fracture: The Diagnostic Challenge

Samia Belfellah, Amina Gharibi, Sihame Chemlali, Nadia Khlil and Jamila Kissa

Abstract

The diagnosis of vertical root fractures (VRFs) is a challenge for dental surgeons because of the similarity of clinical signs with other pathologies. It involves both clinical and radiological examination. Common signs of VRFs are deep localized periodontal pocket, gingival swelling, tenderness to percussion, and radiographic bone loss. The fracture line would be difficult to identify, so an analysis of clinical and radiological data would be required. The use of conservative approaches to avoid tooth extraction is cited in the literature. However, extraction is often unavoidable. The early diagnosis is important because it may avoid unnecessary treatment and excessive bone loss. The aim of this work is to provide more knowledge about the signs and symptoms of vertical root fractures with illustrations by clinical cases.

Keywords: tooth fractures, diagnosis, bone loss, periodontal pocket, extraction

1. Introduction

Root fractures can be classified based on the trajectory of the fracture (vertical, transverse, or oblique), their extent (complete or incomplete), location (apical, midroot, or cervical regions), and the healing/repair mode [1].

Vertical root fractures (VRFs) are defined as longitudinal fractures that might begin on the internal canal wall and extend outward to the external root surface [1].

The fracture is manifested by a partial or total separation of the root substance in the longitudinal axis of the tooth [2].

They develop from the apical or coronal region and extend along the root. They are the third most common cause of extractions of endodontically treated teeth [3]. These fractures may be complete or incomplete and often follow the vestibulo-lingual direction [4].

The incidence of VRF in endodontically treated extracted teeth is 10.9% [5]. In contrast, Yoshino et al. (2015) [6] found that VRFs were the cause of extraction in 31.7% of cases and 93.6% of teeth with endodontic treatment.

The clinical signs associated with VRFs are similar to the clinical signs of failed endodontic treatment or periodontal disease. The delay in diagnosis due to the similarity of clinical signs will direct the treatment plan toward inappropriate therapies (endodontic retreatment, periodontal treatment, apical resection). The difficulty of diagnosis will result in significant bone loss. Hence, it is important to analyze correctly clinical and radiographic data that may be related to VRFs [2, 3].

The aim of this work is to provide more knowledge about the signs and symptoms of vertical fractures with illustrations by clinical cases.

2. Causes of vertical root fractures

The VRFs are usually encountered in restored and/or endodontically treated teeth. They are then defined as "a complication of root canal treatment, characterized by a complete or incomplete fracture initiated from the root at any level, usually directed buccolingually" [7].

In fact, the stress distribution pattern in a tooth restored using post, core, and crown is distinctly dissimilar to that of an intact tooth. The key differences between intact tooth and tooth restored using post-core are:

- occurrence of regions of stress concentration.
- increase in the tensile stresses produced within the remaining tooth structure of a post-core restored tooth [8].

The intensity of stress concentration and tensile stresses will depend upon:

- the material properties of the crown, post, and core material,
- the shape of the post,
- the adhesive strength at the crown-tooth, core-tooth, and core-post, post-tooth interfaces,
- the magnitude and direction of occlusal loads,
- the amount of available tooth structure,
- the anatomy of the tooth [8].

The causes of VRFs would then be [2, 9]: excessive root canal preparation, excessive forces during compaction of the root filling material, excessive root canal enlargement during preparation of the post socket, and internal resorption.

PradeepKumar et al. (2016) [10] reported that 79% of teeth with VRF had dense overfilled root canals. In a recent study [11], it was also found that VRFs were present at a significantly lesser frequency (26%) in roots that were not overfilled.

An isthmus connecting root canals may also promote VRF propagation in the horizontal plane, as it can be considered a naturally weak plane [12].

Endodontic retreatment has also been associated with an increased risk of VRF after 1–8 years of follow-up [13]. Since VRFs appear in teeth with either poor or good quality root canal treatments, VRFs must be considered a potential complication, not necessarily a direct result of a practitioner's procedural error [7].

A recent meta-analysis concluded that filling the canal with Gutta-percha/AH plus does not straighten endodontically treated roots. On the contrary, the Resilon system enhances the resistance of roots to VRF. As this meta-analysis was based on in vitro studies, it should be careful to extrapolate its conclusion to the clinical context [14].

Also, VRFs are encountered in endodontically untreated teeth. They are the apical extension of a coronal fracture. They follow dental fissures secondary to excessive occlusal forces (bruxism) or iatrogenic restorations [15].

There have been some reports of spontaneous VRF, especially in literature from eastern Asia [16].

Yang et al. [17] and Chan et al. [18] reported 12 cases and 64 cases, respectively, of spontaneous VRF in non-endodontically treated teeth. Chan et al. [19] also investigated 315 VRF cases in Chinese patients through a 13-year survey and found that about 40% of all cases occurred in non-endodontically treated teeth.

VRFs are more common in elderly patients. This may be associated with the prevalence of restorations and endodontic treatment with age leading to weakening of the tooth structure. Additionally, as mineral concentration increases with age, the tooth becomes more fragile and may fracture under high load [8, 15].

Premolar and Molar teeth are more prone to fracture than incisors [20]. The prevalence of VRFs is 52% in maxillary and mandibular premolars, followed by the mesial roots of mandibular molars at 24%, maxillary and mandibular central and lateral incisors at 14%, and mesio-vestibular and palatal roots of maxillary molars [21].

3. Diagnostic elements of vertical root fractures

The diagnosis of VRFs is problematic because of the absence of specific clinical (**Figures 1a, 2a, 3a**) and radiographic (**Figures 1b, 2b, 3b–c**) symptoms and signs. Diagnosis therefore relies on invasive techniques including exploratory surgery (**Figures 1d–e, 2c**) [4].

The most common signs of VRF are [2, 22, 23]:

- Deep periodontal pocket bleeding on probing with suppuration.
- Pain on percussion. The patient reports pain on chewing. Pain may be moderate to severe depending on the extent or progression of the lesion.
- The presence of a fistula is a common sign of VRFs. Fistulae are located on the vestibular side and in the most coronal part of the root [2]. The presence of two fistulas (lingual and vestibular) or multiple fistulas is often pathognomonic of VRF [24].

Llena-Puy et al. (2001) [25] concluded in their study of 25 cases of vertical fractures that periodontal pocketing and diffuse pain are the most common signs of VRF. Tamse et al. (1999) [26], in a sample of 92 cases of vertical fractures, found a periodontal pocket in 67% of cases, pain in 55% of cases, and sensitivity to percussion in 33% of cases. These authors stated that the fistula when it exists is located close to the marginal gingiva. Cohen et al. (2006) [27] found that pain on percussion was present in 69.74% of cases, pain on chewing in 61.74% of cases, and swelling and fistulation were present in only 15.35 and 18.42%, respectively. In a study by Karygianni et al. (2014) [28], the presence of a deep periodontal pocket existed in only 24% of cases.

See et al. (2019) [29] found that the clinical signs most associated with VRF are: the presence of a fistula, a periodontal pocket ≥5 mm, abscess or swelling at the periodontium, and the J-shaped or clear halot image on radiographic examination.

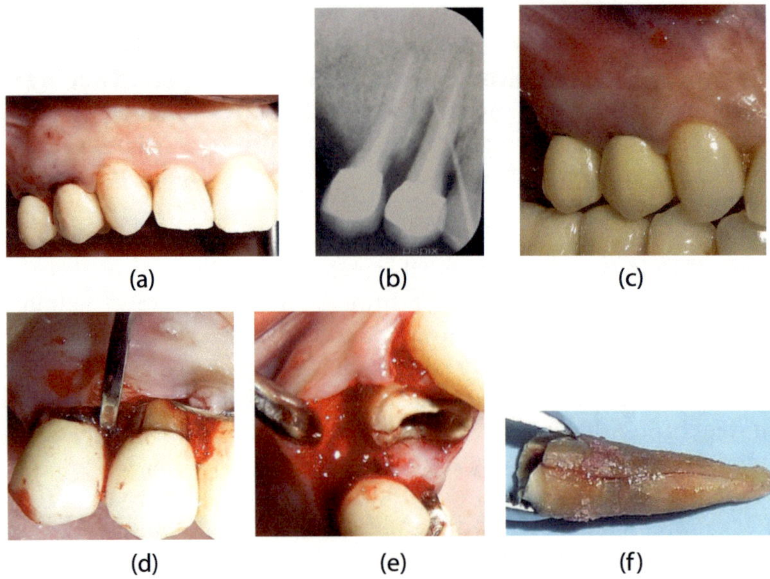

Figure 1.
(a) Initial clinical view showing swelling and fistula in relation to 14. Wear facets are present on the lower incisors; (b) Retro-alveolar radiograph with gutta cone in the fistula showing: - Lateral root radiolucency distal to 14; – Desmodontal enlargement; – The gutta cone stops lateral to the root at the apical 1/3; (c) Clinical view at 4 weeks. There is a reduction in swelling with the persistence of the bleeding pocket distal to 14; (d) An exploratory flap was then performed and revealed a vertical fracture line distal to 14; (e) After removal of the crown, the fracture extends to the inner surface of the post; and (f) The fracture line extends vertically across the root.

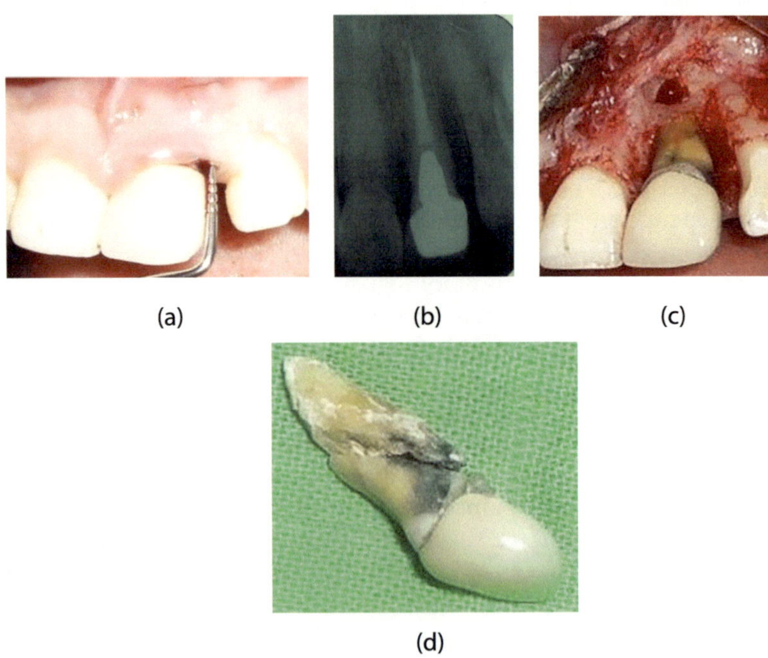

Figure 2.
(a) 5 mm deep pocket distal to 21; (b) Retro-alveolar radiograph showing a marginal bone loss in the tooth 21 and an excess in filling material with a slight periapical reaction; (c) Flap elevation surgery showing vestibular and proximal bone loss on the 21; and (d) Extraction of the tooth. A vertical fracture in the mesio-distal direction was identified.

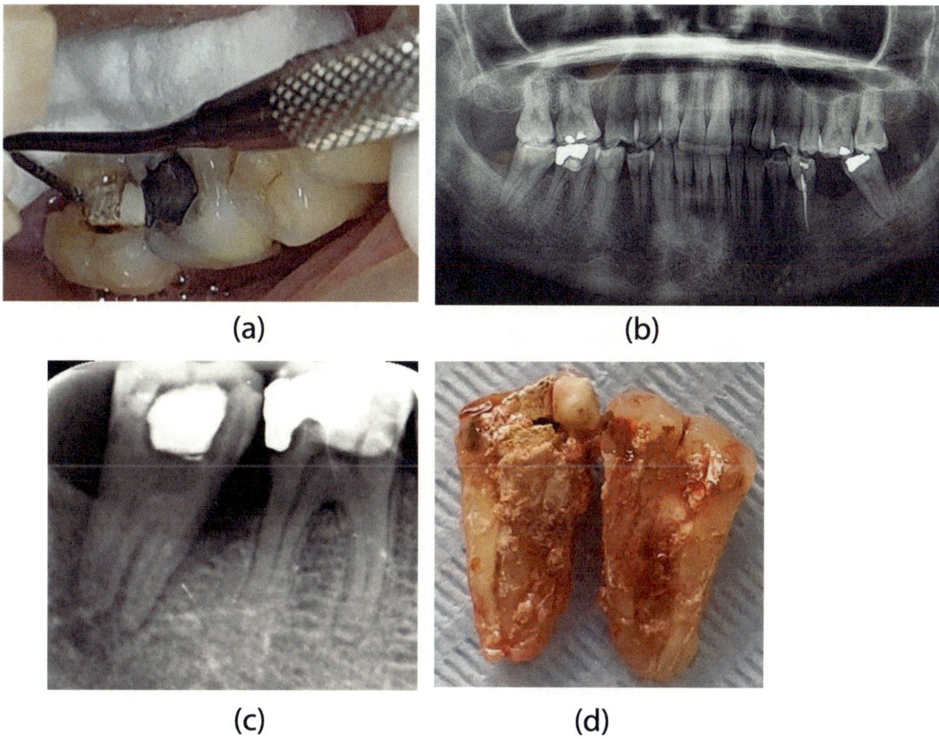

Figure 3.
(a) Initial view showing decay and coronal fracture of 47; (b) Panoramic radiograph showing generalized chronic periodontitis; (c) Retro-alveolar radiograph showing: - Insufficient coronal radiopacity (weakened tooth structure); – Deep bone lysis; – Root canal enlargement of the distal root; – Enlargement of the periodontal ligament; – The fracture line visualized in the coronal portion of the tooth; and (d) Dental extraction of the 47. We can note the infiltration of granulomatous tissue inside of the fracture line.

On radiographic examination, we note [21, 30]:

- "Halot appearance" in the form of peri-radicular and periapical radiolucency.
- Angular radiolucency extending from the bony ridge laterally to the root.
- Presence of furcation involvement at the pluriradicular level.
- Diffuse desmodontal enlargement.

Periapical radiography can detect the fracture line in only 35.7% of cases because of the superposition of the fracture line with the root canals or the dental roots or the non-parallelism of the X-ray beam with the fracture plane [3].

The cone beam and conventional tomography (CBCT) allow the visualization of the fracture line. However, their high cost limits their use [21]. The studies that have confirmed the superiority of this type of radiography over conventional radiography are in vitro studies [31], the clinical interpretation of these results is different [32].

The presence of metal in the root canal and the voxel size in the CBCT setting significantly interfere with the radiological diagnosis of VRFs. The use of filters does not reduce the artifact caused by metal posts. For mesio-distal vertical fractures, the CBCT image remains better than the periapical radiograph [33].

There is a lack of evidence supporting the superiority of cone beam radiography over conventional radiography in the diagnosis of VRFs [32]. Baageel et al. (2016) [34] concluded in their systematic review that CBCT radiography is the technique of choice for the detection of vertical fractures in VRF. In contrast, a recent systematic review of the literature showed that CBCT radiography is still not a good means of diagnosing VRFs in root canal-filled teeth compared to direct visualization [35].

Digital subtraction radiography has also proven to be effective in the diagnosis of VRF [36]. The convolutional neural network learning model has also been defined as a promised tool to detect VRFs on panoramic images and to function as a computer-assisted detection/diagnosis system [37].

4. Bone loss secondary to vertical fracture

The fracture is a long apical foramen communicating with spaces that contain profound irritants that generate an immune/inflammatory response that significantly damages the supporting periodontium [38].

The presence of a VRF results in communication between a potentially infected pulp, the periodontal ligament, and the gingival sulcus. Various irritants (bacteria, necrotic pulp tissue, sealants) will enter the fracture line during mastication [3]. In addition, the presence of the fracture line causes irritation of the periodontal ligament leading to diffusion of inflammation and bone loss.

The VRF may evolve into a total division of the tooth. The resulting bone loss will increase in width and depth [4].

Lustig et al. (2000) [30] found that in most patients with clinical signs (fistula, large bone defect, mobility), or with an acute exacerbation, greater proximal bone loss was noted than in patients diagnosed early.

The pattern of bone destruction following VRF has been studied in a case series. It is illustrated in **Figure 4** [39].

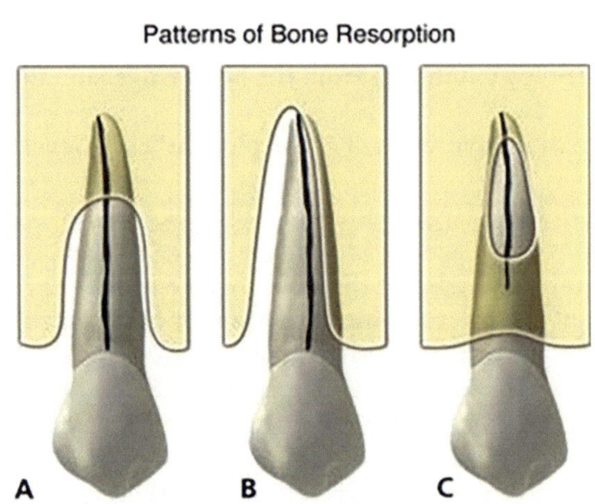

Figure 4.
Patterns of bone destruction [39]. The punch-out defect may extend over part of the root height (A) or to the apex (B) or be in the form of a fenestration (C).

5. Clinical management

Following the diagnosis of root fracture, the decision to preserve or to extract the fractured tooth or root and substitute it with a dental implant is a big dilemma [40]. Traditionally, it was believed that an early decision to extract the tooth is important because the resulting inflammation in the surrounding periodontal apparatus may lead to periodontal breakdown followed by the development of significant osseous destruction [40, 41]. As a result, future dental implant rehabilitation in the area may be compromised [7, 23, 40]. However, each case should be judged objectively as some data revealed that with adequate case selection, proper management of vertical root fractured teeth has no detrimental effect on periodontal tissue [42].

The decision to preserve a tooth with VRF by additional endodontic treatments should rely not only on the technical feasibility of treating the fracture but also on a wider spectrum of periodontal, prosthetic, and esthetic considerations that affect the risk of complications and the long-term prognosis of the tooth [7, 43].

Extraction of the tooth with VRF is usually the treatment of choice (**Figures 1f, 2d, 3d**). Although maintaining a tooth with VRF is crucial for the benefit of the patient, several treatment alternatives can be considered, including root amputation or hemisection [23], a replantation procedure, or flap elevation and sealing of the fracture line [7, 44]. Okaguchi et al. [45] have successfully treated cases of complete VRFs by reimplantation combined with bonding with 4-META/MMA-TBB resin. A case of VRF successfully treated with up to 2 years follow-up was reported in the literature. The treatment option used Biodentine, a bonding agent, a fiber post, and dual-cure resin cement without tooth extraction, followed by a ceramic crown [46].

These unique treatment attempts are based mostly on case reports [47, 48]. Additional large-scale clinical studies are required in order to better define the exact indications, protocols, and expected prognosis of these novel treatments [7]. However, the prognosis is often poor (**Figures 1f, 2d, 3d**) [4, 49].

6. Conclusion

In general, fractures were included as one of the causes of root damage and can result in non periodontal induced abscess [50]. The VRFs are often difficult to diagnose, due to the associated symptoms that are common to endodontic or periodontal damage. Only the confrontation of clinical and radiological data can confirm the diagnosis. In case of doubt, exploratory surgery would be necessary. Despite the therapeutic proposals, extraction of the fractured tooth is often the rule. The early diagnosis of VRFs allows to avoid the bone loss associated with the fracture and the management of this bone loss would be necessary in case of implant placement at the extraction site.

7. Clinical case

7.1 Case N 1

Patient T.H, 49 years old, was referred from the denture department to the periodontal department for a recurrent abscess in the crowned 14.

The clinical examination revealed a swelling with a fistula in front of the 14, a deep localized disto-buccal pocket (8 mm) in the same tooth, and wear facets on the lower incisors.

Radiographic examination revealed bone lysis in the disto-lateral aspect of the root.

After drainage of the abscess, root planning of the pocket in distal of 14, and prescription of amoxicillin-based antibiotics, the patient reported a reduction in clinical signs and the abscess disappearance. However, the persistence of the deep and bleeding pocket distal to the 14 indicated an exploratory flap, which revealed the root fracture line (**Figure 1a–f**).

7.2 Case N 2

Patient E. H, 23 years old, was referred by her dentist for recurrent fistulas and abscesses related to the 21 crown and post-support. Clinical examination revealed multiple fistulas at the level of the attached gingiva and the muco-gingival line in relation to the tooth, a deep localized disto-buccal pocket (5 mm), and a gingival recession of 2 mm in the same localization.

Radiographic examination revealed an exceeding of root canal filling material.

The patient's management began with periodontal pocket planning distal to 21. However, the symptomatology recurred during follow-up sessions. An apical resection was subsequently scheduled to remove the exceeding Gutta. However, the excessive mobility (grade 4) of the tooth during the surgery revealed a fracture in the mesio-distal direction not visible on radiography. The delayed diagnosis of the fracture line resulted in a great osseous defect in the buccal aspect of the tooth (**Figure 2a–d**).

7.3 Case N 3

The patient R. K., aged 40 years, was referred for mobility of the 47.

Clinical examination showed a high mobility of the tooth (grade 3), occlusal temporary filling, and deep pocketing surrounding the tooth (7 mm).

A panoramic radiograph showed a generalized chronic periodontitis. A periapical radiograph revealed deep lysis of the alveolar bone, insufficient coronal radiopacity, and an enlarged endodontic canal of the distal root on 47.

Case management consisted of tooth extraction which objectified the fracture (**Figure 3a–d**).

Acknowledgements

Our acknowledgment goes to all those who contributed to this document.

Conflicts of interest statements

There is no conflict of interest affecting any author.

Disclosure

The clinical case N1 was presented as a poster at EuroPerio8, in June 2015.

DOI: http://dx.doi.org/10.5772/intechopen.1006980

Author details

Samia Belfellah*, Amina Gharibi, Sihame Chemlali, Nadia Khlil and Jamila Kissa
Faculty of Dentistry, Department of Periodontics, University Hassan II of Casablanca, Casablanca, Morocco

*Address all correspondence to: belfellahsamia@yahoo.fr

References

[1] Ercoli C, Caton JG. Dental prostheses and tooth-related factors. Journal of Clinical Periodontology. 2018;**45**(Suppl. 20):S207-S218

[2] von Arx T, Bosshardt D. Vertical root fractures of endodontically treated posterior teeth: A histologic analysis with clinical and radiographic correlates. Swiss Dental Journal. 2017;**127**(1):14-23

[3] Khasnis SA, Kidiyoor KH, Patil AB, Kenganal SB. Vertical root fractures and their management. Journal of Conservative Dentistry. 2014;**17**(2):103-110

[4] Corbella S, Tamse A, Nemcovsky C, Taschieri S. Diagnostic issues dealing with the management of teeth with vertical root fractures: A narrative review. Giornale Italiano di Endodonzia. 2014;**28**(2):91-96

[5] Fuss Z, Lustig J, Tamse A. Prevalence of vertical root fractures in extracted endodontically treated teeth. International Endodontic Journal. 1999;**32**(4):283-286

[6] Yoshino K, Ito K, Kuroda M, Sugihara N. Prevalence of vertical root fracture as the reason for tooth extraction in dental clinics. Clinical Oral Investigations. 2015;**19**(6):1405-1409

[7] Tsesis I, Beitlitum I, Rosen E. Treatment alternatives for the preservation of vertically root fractured teeth. In: Tamse A, Tsesis I, Rosen E, editors. Vertical Root Fractures in Dentistry. Cham: Springer; 2015. pp. 97-107

[8] Kishen A. Mechanisms and risk factors for fracture predilection in endodontically treated teeth. Endodontic Topics. 2006;**13**(1):57-83

[9] Martins JNR, Canta JP, Coelho A, Baharestani M. Vertical root fracture diagnosis of crowned premolars with root canal treatment – Two case reports. Revista Portuguesa de Estomatologia, Medicina Dentária e Cirurgia Maxilofacial. 2014;**55**(1):60-64

[10] PradeepKumar AR, Shemesh H, Jothilatha S, Vijayabharathi R, Jayalakshmi S, Kishen A. Diagnosis of vertical root fractures in restored Endodontically treated teeth: A time-dependent retrospective cohort study. Journal of Endodontics. 2016;**42**(8):1175-1180

[11] PradeepKumar AR, Shemesh H, van Loveren C, JothiLatha S, Shireen F, VijayaBharathi R, et al. Impact of apical extent of root canal filling on vertical root fracture: A case–control study. International Endodontic Journal. 2019;**52**(9):1283-1289

[12] Chai H, Tamse A. The effect of isthmus on vertical root fracture in Endodontically treated teeth. Journal of Endodontics. 2015;**41**(9):1515-1519

[13] García-Guerrero C, Parra-Junco C, Quijano-Guauque S, Molano N, Pineda GA, Marín-Zuluaga DJ. Vertical root fractures in endodontically-treated teeth: A retrospective analysis of possible risk factors. Journal of Investigative and Clinical Dentistry. 2018;**9**(1):e12273

[14] Tan M, Chai Z, Sun C, Hu B, Gao X, Chen Y, et al. Comparative evaluation of the vertical fracture resistance of endodontically treated roots filled with Gutta-percha and Resilon: A meta-analysis of in vitro studies. BMC Oral Health. 2018;**18**(1):107

[15] Bhaskar U, Logani A, Shah N. True vertical tooth root fracture: Case report

and review. Contemporary Clinical Dentistry. 2011;**2**(3):265-268

[16] Lim MJ, Kim JA, Choi Y, Hong CU, Min KS. Differentiating spontaneous vertical root fracture in endodontically treated tooth. European Journal of Dentistry. 2017;**11**(01):122-125

[17] Yang SF, Rivera EM, Walton RE. Vertical root fracture in nonendodontically treated teeth. Journal of Endodontics. 1995;**21**(6):337-339

[18] Chan CP, Tseng SC, Lin CP, Huang CC, Tsai TP, Chen CC. Vertical root fracture in nonendodontically treated teeth –A clinical report of 64 cases in Chinese patients. Journal of Endodontics. 1998;**24**(10):678-681

[19] Chan CP, Lin CP, Tseng SC, Jeng JH. Vertical root fracture in endodontically versus nonendodontically treated teeth: A survey of 315 cases in Chinese patients. Oral Surgery, Oral Medicine, Oral Pathology, Oral Radiology, and Endodontology. 1999;**87**(4):504-507

[20] Hsiao LT, Ho JC, Huang CF, Hung WC, Chang CW. Analysis of clinical associated factors of vertical root fracture cases found in endodontic surgery. Journal of Dental Sciences. 2020;**15**(2):200-206

[21] Freitas PQ, Rabêlo-Júnior PMS, Alves CMC, Souza S. de FC. The diagnostic challenge of vertical root fracture in endodontically treated teeth: A case report. Revista Odonto Ciência. 2012;**27**(1):82-86

[22] Oya EO, Pallos D, Schwartz-Filho HO, Brandt WC, Sendyk WR, Roman-Torres CV. Vertical root fracture: Preservation of the alveolar ridge using immediate implants. Case Reports in Dentistry. 2014;**2014**(520169):1-6

[23] Tamse A. Vertical root fractures in endodontically treated teeth: Diagnostic signs and clinical management. Endodontic Topics. 2006;**13**(1):84-94

[24] Chandhana D, Saipavithra R. A review on vertical root fracture. Journal of Pharmaceutical Sciences. 2015;7(6):387-389

[25] Llena-Puy MC, Forner-Navarro L, Barbero-Navarro I. Vertical root fracture in endodontically treated teeth: A review of 25 cases. Oral Surgery, Oral Medicine, Oral Pathology, Oral Radiology, and Endodontology. 2001;**92**(5):553-555

[26] Tamse A, Fuss Z, Lustig J, Kaplavi J. An evaluation of endodontically treated vertically fractured teeth. Journal of Endodontics. 1999;**25**(7):506-508

[27] Cohen S, Berman LH, Blanco L, Bakland LK, Kim JS. A demographic analysis of vertical root fractures. Journal of Endodontics. 2006;**32**(12):1160-1163

[28] Karygianni L, Krengel M, Winter M, Stampf S, Wrbas KT. Comparative assessment of the incidence of vertical root fractures between conventional versus surgical endodontic retreatment. Clinical Oral Investigations. 2014;**18**(8):2015-2021

[29] See WK, Ho JC, Huang CF, Hung WC, Chang CW. The association between clinical diagnostic factors and the prevalence of vertical root fracture in endodontic surgery. Journal of the Formosan Medical Association. 2019;**118**(3):713-720

[30] Lustig JP, Tamse A, Fuss Z. Pattern of bone resorption in vertically fractured, endodontically treated teeth. Oral Surgery, Oral Medicine, Oral Pathology, Oral Radiology, and Endodontology. 2000;**90**(2):224-227

[31] Al Hadi D, Parekh S, Naeem W, Luke AM, Mathew S. Detection of vertical root fractures using three different imaging modalities: An In vitro study. The Journal of Contemporary Dental Practice. 2020;**21**(5):549-553

[32] Corbella S, Del Fabbro M, Tamse A, Rosen E, Tsesis I, Taschieri S. Cone beam computed tomography for the diagnosis of vertical root fractures: A systematic review of the literature and meta-analysis. Oral Surgery, Oral Medicine, Oral Pathology and Oral Radiology. 2014;**118**(5):593-602

[33] De Martin E Silva D, Campos CN, Pires Carvalho AC, Devito KL. Diagnosis of Mesiodistal vertical root fractures in teeth with metal posts: Influence of applying filters in cone-beam computed tomography images at different resolutions. Journal of Endodontics. 2018;**44**(3):470-474

[34] Baageel TM, Allah EH, Bakalka G, Jadu F, Yamany I, Jan AM, et al. Vertical root fracture: Biological effects and accuracy of diagnostic imaging methods. Journal of International Society of Preventive & Community Dentistry. 2016;**6**(Suppl 2):S93-S104

[35] PradeepKumar AR, Shemesh H, Nivedhitha MS, Hashir MMJ, Arockiam S, Uma Maheswari TN, et al. Diagnosis of vertical root fractures by cone-beam computed tomography in root-filled teeth with confirmation by direct visualization: A systematic review and meta-analysis. Journal of Endodontics. 2021;**47**(8):1198-1214

[36] Mikrogeorgis G, Eirinaki E, Kapralos V, Koutroulis A, Lyroudia K, Pitas I. Diagnosis of vertical root fractures in endodontically treated teeth utilising digital subtraction radiography: A case series report. Australian Endodontic Journal. 2018;**44**(3):286-291

[37] Fukuda M, Inamoto K, Shibata N, Ariji Y, Yanashita Y, Kutsuna S, et al. Evaluation of an artificial intelligence system for detecting vertical root fracture on panoramic radiography. Oral Radiology. 2020;**36**(4):337-343

[38] Walton RE, Rivera E. Pathogenesis of the vertical root fracture. In: Tamse A, Tsesis I, Rosen E, editors. Vertical Root Fractures in Dentistry. Cham: Springer; 2015. pp. 87-96

[39] Walton RE. Vertical root fracture : Factors related to identification. The Journal of the American Dental Association. 2017;**148**(2):100-105

[40] Tsesis I, Rosen E, Tamse A, Taschieri S, Kfir A. Diagnosis of vertical root fractures in Endodontically treated teeth based on clinical and radiographic indices: A systematic review. Journal of Endodontics. 2010;**36**(9):1455-1458

[41] Walton RE, Michelich RJ, Smith GN. The histopathogenesis of vertical root fractures. Journal of Endodontics. 1984;**10**(2):48-56

[42] Eichelsbacher F, Denner W, Klaiber B, Schlagenhauf U. Periodontal status of teeth with crown-root fractures: Results two years after adhesive fragment reattachment. Journal of Clinical Periodontology. 2009;**36**(10):905-911

[43] Sim IGB, Lim TS, Krishnaswamy G, Chen NN. Decision making for retention of Endodontically treated posterior cracked teeth: A 5-year follow-up study. Journal of Endodontics. 2016;**42**(2):225-229

[44] Sugaya T, Tomita M, Motoki Y, Miyaji H, Kawamami M. Influence of enamel matrix derivative on healing of root surfaces after bonding treatment and intentional replantation of vertically fractured roots. Dental Traumatology. 2016;**32**(5):397-401

[45] Okaguchi M, Kuo T, Ho YC. Successful treatment of vertical root fracture through intentional replantation and root fragment bonding with 4-META/MMA-TBB resin. Journal of the Formosan Medical Association. 2019;**118**(3):671-678

[46] Baranwal HC, Singh N, Kumar N, Garg R, Yadav J, Tripathi R. New approach in the Management of Vertical Root Fracture with the help of biodentine and CBCT. Case Reports in Dentistry. 2020;**2020**:1-6

[47] Taschieri S, Tamse A, Del Fabbro M, Rosano G, Tsesis I. A new surgical technique for preservation of endodontically treated teeth with coronally located vertical root fractures: A prospective case series. Oral Surgery, Oral Medicine, Oral Pathology, Oral Radiology, and Endodontology. 2010;**110**(6):e45-e52

[48] Floratos SG, Kratchman SI. Surgical Management of Vertical Root Fractures for posterior teeth: Report of four cases. Journal of Endodontics. 2012;**38**(4):550-555

[49] Hadrossek PH, Dammaschke T. New treatment option for an incomplete vertical root fracture–a preliminary case report. Head & Face Medicine. 2014;**10**(1):9

[50] Herrera D, Retamal-Valdes B, Alonso B, Feres M. Acute periodontal lesions (periodontal abscesses and necrotizing periodontal diseases) and endo-periodontal lesions. Journal of Clinical Periodontology. 2018;**45**(S20):S78-S94

Chapter 3

Dental Trauma and Association with Periodontium

Kumari Abhilasha

Abstract

Dental trauma is an unexpected and unfortunate event that can cause varying degrees of damage to the teeth and often leaves a lasting psychological impact. This chapter deals in brief about different types of dental trauma, how periodontal health maintains the integrity of teeth, and the factors that predispose individuals to trauma, including the biomechanical mechanisms involved. Additionally, the chapter explores the responses of both healthy and diseased periodontium to trauma, emphasizing that a healthy periodontium not only resists sudden damage but also supports faster recovery. Conclusively focusing on the management and implication of digitization and artificial intelligence in dental traumas, which determines the prognosis and longevity of the treated tooth.

Keywords: dental trauma, WHO classification, risk factors, biomechanism of trauma, healthy and diseased periodontal response, management, artificial intelligence

1. Introduction

Dental trauma refers to the injury sustained by a tooth and its supporting structures due to the sudden impact of energy. It can result in fractures, displacement, or even loss of the tooth, negatively affecting function, esthetics, and the individual's psychological well-being. Due to the associated physical and emotional damage, it presents one of the most challenging situations for a dentist to manage. When a patient visits the outpatient area with a traumatic dental injury (TDI), it should be treated as a dental emergency, and immediate first aid should be administered.

Any injury to the teeth, whether primary or permanent, can affect the enamel, dentin, pulp, and the surrounding periodontium. The ability of the periodontium to heal depends on systemic health along with the periodontal condition of the affected tooth or teeth. A healthy periodontium typically responds well to external forces through adaptive bone remodeling. In contrast, teeth with compromised periodontal health are more susceptible to severe damage from external impacts, leading to compromised healing responses.

Dental trauma impacts physical health and psychological well-being, causing compromised oral health-related quality of life. Therefore, it is essential that not only the attending dentist but also parents, teachers, and care providers possess basic knowledge about immediate management. The success of treatment largely depends on the level of expertise and understanding of the injuries and their management.

2. Classification of dental trauma

Classification is crucial for the quantitative analysis of any phenomenon and plays a vital role in enhancing communication among individuals [1].

In the 1950s, pediatric dentist G.E. Ellis pioneered the promotion of a universal classification of dental injuries to carry out the treatment plan swiftly toward patient well-being. Since then, various classifications have been proposed for TDI [2]. The following outlines the classification provided by the World Health Organization (WHO) (**Table 1**) [3, 4].

To enhance data sharing and comparability with clinical datasets, the International Classification of Diseases published by the WHO can also be utilized for recording trauma [5]. However, even being quite elaborate in description, there are still certain conditions that one comes up with in daily clinical practice that do not fit into the classification, namely-

a. ONLY pulp injury without enamel, dentin, and cementum involvement with loss of vitality.

b. ONLY pulp injury without enamel, dentin, and cementum involvement without loss of vitality.

c. Untreated long-term non-vital asymptomatic tooth.

Type of injury (code according to WHO)	
Injuries to the hard-dental tissues and the pulp	Description
Enamel infraction (N 502.50)	An incomplete fracture (crack) of the enamel without loss of tooth substance.
Enamel fracture (N 502.50)	A fracture with loss of tooth substance confined to the enamel.
Enamel-dentin fracture (N 502.51)	A fracture with loss of tooth substance confined to enamel and dentin but not involving the pulp.
Complicated crown fracture (N 502.52)	A fracture involving enamel and dentin and exposing the pulp.
Uncomplicated crown-root fracture (N 502.54)	A fracture involving enamel, dentin and cementum, but not exposing the pulp.
Complicated crown-root fracture (N 502.54)	A fracture involving enamel, dentin, and cementum and exposing the pulp.
Root fracture (N 502.53)	A fracture involving dentin, cementum, and the pulp.
Injuries to the periodontal tissues	
Concussion (N 503.20)	No abnormal loosening or displacement of the tooth, but marked reaction to percussion.
Subluxation [Loosening] (N 503.20)	Abnormal loosening, but without displacement of the tooth.
Extrusive luxation [Peripheral dislocation, Partial avulsion] (N 503.20)	Partial displacement of the tooth out of its socket.
Lateral luxation (N 503.20)	Displacement of the tooth in a direction other than axially.

Type of injury (code according to WHO)	
Intrusive luxation [central dislocation] (N 503.21)	Displacement of the tooth into the alveolar bone.
Avulsion [Exarticulation] (N 503.22)	Complete displacement of the tooth out of its socket.
Injuries to supporting bone	
Comminution of the maxillary alveolar socket (N 502.40)	Crushing and compression of the alveolar socket.
Comminution of the mandibular alveolar socket (N 502.60)	
Fracture of the maxillary alveolar socket (N 502.40)	A fracture confined to the facial or oral socket wall.
Fracture of the mandibular alveolar socket (N 502.60)	
Fracture of the maxillary alveolar process (N 502.40)	A fracture of the alveolar process, which may or may not involve the alveolar socket.
Fracture of the mandibular alveolar process (N 502.60)	
Fracture of the maxillae (N 502.42)	A fracture involving the base of the maxilla or mandible and often the alveolar process (jaw fracture). The fracture may or may not involve the alveolar socket.
Fracture of the mandible (N 502.61)	
Injuries to gingiva or oral mucosa	
Laceration of gingiva or oral mucosa (S 01.50)	A shallow or deep wound in the mucosa resulting from a tear and usually produced by a sharp object.
Contusion of gingiva or oral mucosa (S 00.50)	A bruise usually produced by impact with a blunt object and no break in the mucosa.
Abrasion of gingiva or oral mucosa (S 00.50)	A superficial wound produced by rubbing or scraping of the mucosa, leaving a raw, bleeding surface.

Table 1.
WHO classification of dental injury.

3. Factors affecting the stage of damage and association with PDL

It's crucial to keep in mind that trauma arises both from external and internal influences and can stem from various factors. The relevance of these factors determines the extent of damage exerted. These factors can be divided into two types: Extrinsic factors and intrinsic factors. Extrinsic factors comprise the conditions outside the oral cavity that influence the severity of injury due to dental trauma. Intrinsic factors relate to the teeth and oral environment that determine the effect and response to the trauma (**Table 2**).

3.1 Extrinsic factors

3.1.1 Energy of impact/fall

Generally speaking, dental traumas occur due to collisions that generate significant force, leading to injuries [6]. This factor includes both mass and velocity. Velocity plays a greater role since energy is the result of mass times the square of velocity ($E = mc^2$) [7].

Extrinsic factors	Intrinsic factors
1. Energy of Impact/Fall	1. Type of Dentition
2. Resilience of impacting object	2. Biological aspect of teeth
3. Shape of impacting object	3. Anatomical aspect of teeth
4. Direction of impact	4. Occlusion

Table 2.
Extrinsic and intrinsic factors.

Low-velocity blows cause the greatest damage to the supporting structures that include periodontal ligament fiber, gingival fiber, and alveolar bone, whereas tooth fractures are less pronounced. In contrast, in high-velocity impacts, the energy of the impact is apparently expended in creating the fracture and is seldom transmitted to any great extent to the root or supporting structures of the tooth [4].

Hence, the energy of impact is an important variable causing the extent of trauma to the tooth and associated structures.

3.1.2 Resilience of impacting object

The hardness or softness of the impacting object also influences the severity of the injury, even when the impact energy is the same. Hitting the teeth against a hard surface involves a great mass and low velocity, but because of the non-resilience of the surface, the energy will not be distributed as much, giving a sharper force which favors hard tissue injuries and fewer teeth injured simultaneously [8].

Hitting the teeth against a resilient surface often results in periodontal tissue injuries of several teeth simultaneously. This is because a low-velocity impact with a resilient surface can distribute the energy across several teeth, allowing them time to adapt to the force and transmit it more gradually to the healthy periodontal tissues; hence, the chance of crown fracture is reduced while the risk of luxation and alveolar fracture is increased [4, 7].

Soft tissues like lips and cheeks and mouthguards provide resilience, and impact can be dampened by them as they come between teeth and an impacting object, causing absorption of energy and distribution to several teeth with more periodontal tissue damage [7].

3.1.3 Shape of impacting object

The shape of the impacting object is also crucial in determining the extent of damage. A sharp object will have a smaller contact area, leading to less energy distribution and a higher likelihood of causing a fracture at the point of contact. However, a blunt object will have larger surface area contact, which will distribute the force to the periodontal tissues, causing more trauma to the periodontium. In the case of healthy periodontium, the resistance will transmit the forces to the apical region of the tooth, causing more chances of root fracture or avulsion [7].

3.1.4 Direction of impact

The direction of the force significantly influences how fracture lines spread. The impact can meet the tooth at different angles, most often hitting the tooth facially and perpendicular to the long axis of the root. Fractures like cervical crown fractures, oblique crown-root fractures, and oblique root fractures are seen when horizontal force is exerted on the labial surface of the tooth. On the other hand, vertical impact force tends to cause crazing lines limited to the cervical portion of enamel and cementum [9].

3.2 Intrinsic factors

3.2.1 Type of dentition

The type of dentition during trauma also influences the tissue's response. Trauma occurring during primary dentition can significantly impact the developing permanent teeth. Injuries to primary teeth have more impact on periodontal tissue. Because the apex of primary teeth is close to the bud of the permanent teeth, damage to primary dentition can affect the eruption of permanent teeth. The severity of these effects depends on the patient's age, the degree of root resorption, and the type and extent of the trauma [10].

Injury to the dental follicle can result in damage to the follicle itself and increase the likelihood of ankylosis between the tooth surface and the crypt, potentially halting the eruption process [4].

Injuries are frequently observed during the mixed dentition period. Environmental factors and activities, such as cycling, skateboarding, and falls during play, are major contributors to trauma. Injuries during this stage can affect teeth with incomplete root development, potentially leading to pulp devitalization [11].

Additionally, such injuries can disrupt tooth alignment due to premature loss of teeth and damage to periodontal ligament fibers.

3.2.2 Biological aspect of teeth

a. *Stage of root development*-The stage of root development is a key prognostic factor in predicting pulp healing [12]. When the root is not fully developed, there is a higher likelihood of pulp revascularization, and root development can continue. However, if trauma is not treated and remains unaddressed for an extended period, pulp necrosis may occur, especially in cases with irregularly shaped canals. For teeth with fully formed roots, the risk of bacterial invasion is greater, which hinders pulp revascularization and leads to pulp necrosis [7].

Marginal bone loss is notably affected by the stage of root development. In teeth with immature roots, marginal bone loss and repair-related replacement root resorption are significantly less common compared to teeth with fully developed roots [13]. This is because the alveolar bone around immature teeth is less mineralized and more resilient, providing a shock-absorbing effect to traumatic impacts [7].

b. *Shape of root formation*-Teeth with flared roots have more interdental bone and better anchorage than those with fused or convergent roots. The impact on teeth with divergent roots is distributed evenly. However, teeth with convergent roots are more prone to luxation from even minor impacts, as the force distribution to the supporting structure is reduced and absorbed more by the tooth itself. Conditions such as dilacerated roots have a higher likelihood of fracturing at the apex.

c. *Degree of tooth displacement*-The degree of tooth displacement within the alveolar socket is a crucial factor influencing the healing of both the pulp and periodontal tissues. Teeth with minimal or no displacement generally have a better prognosis, as there is less damage to the neurovascular bundle, cementum, and PDL. Conversely, displaced teeth face a higher risk of damaging the marginal alveolar bone and surrounding gingival tissue, leading to increased marginal periodontal breakdown [7].

d. *Extent of pulp involvement*-Extensive involvement of the pulp can compromise the neurovascular supply, which in turn can impair tissue healing and function, potentially resulting in root fracture healing with connective tissue and internal inflammatory root resorption. Young pulps are more resilient and can survive even with significant traumatic exposure and prolonged exposure time, provided there is no accompanying luxation injury.

3.2.3 Anatomical aspect of teeth

Certain anatomical variations or malalignments can increase the risk of frequent dental trauma. Factors such as bimaxillary protrusion, Class 2 Division 1 malocclusion, large overjet (> 3 mm), incompetent lips, and mouth breathing can predispose individuals to dental injuries (**Figure 1**) [14]. Individuals with an overjet greater than 3 mm are more susceptible to direct impact on their teeth during accidents [3]. Similarly, those with incompetent lips lack the protective cushioning provided by the lips, resulting in direct impact on the teeth. This direct force often affects individual teeth, increasing the likelihood of dentoalveolar fractures. Additionally, the labial protrusion of teeth reduces the thickness of the buccal or labial bony plate, which decreases its ability to absorb and transmit force effectively.

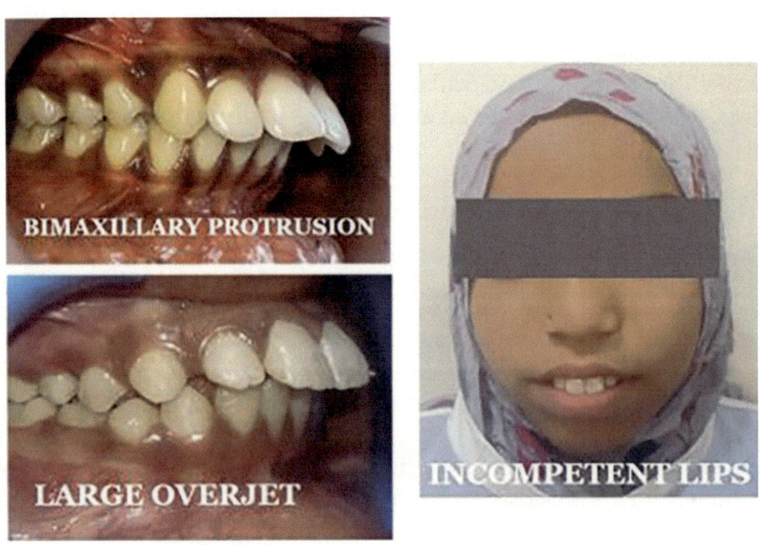

Figure 1.
Anatomical risk factors.

3.2.4 Occlusion

Any trauma experienced by teeth due to occlusion has been termed trauma from occlusion. Trauma from occlusion is defined as an injury to the attachment apparatus as a result of excessive occlusal forces. The etiology of occlusion-related trauma includes the orientation of the teeth's long axis in relation to the forces to which they are subjected, the morphology of the roots, and the morphology of the alveolar process, plaque, the fabrication of long span bridges on a few teeth, injudicious bone resection during surgical procedures, parafunctional habits, food impaction, overhanging fillings, poorly contoured crowns and bridges, and ill-fitting dentures [15].

This clinical condition is frequently associated with jiggling forces and results in an increasing or progressive tooth mobility [16].

4. Biomechanism of trauma

While direct forces are the most prevalent, understanding how impact is distributed during oblique dental trauma is crucial for fully grasping the biomechanics of dentoalveolar trauma and its effects on periodontal structures.

4.1 External impact forces

If a tooth experiences a labial horizontal impact greater than the resisting force of the periodontal ligament (PDL) tissues, the resulting trauma can cause compressive forces on the enamel, leading to the splitting of enamel rods. This impact then distributes toward the lingual side and reaches the dentino-enamel junction (DEJ), where most of the crack's energy is dissipated (**Figure 2**) [4, 9, 17]. The DEJ is 5–10 times tougher than enamel but 75% less tough than dentin [18]. Due to enamel's brittleness and dentin's greater toughness, the DEJ resists crack propagation [19]. It can absorb a significant amount of force, potentially arresting the crack before it propagates into the dentin [17]. However, if the impact force exceeds the DEJ's resistance, the crack can advance into the dentin, resulting in a horizontal fracture of the crown (**Figure 3**).

When teeth experience an oblique impact, high stresses initially concentrate at the impact site and subsequently propagate toward the root apex, which is also seen in the finite element analysis (FEA) study by Jayasudha et al. [9] (**Figure 4**).

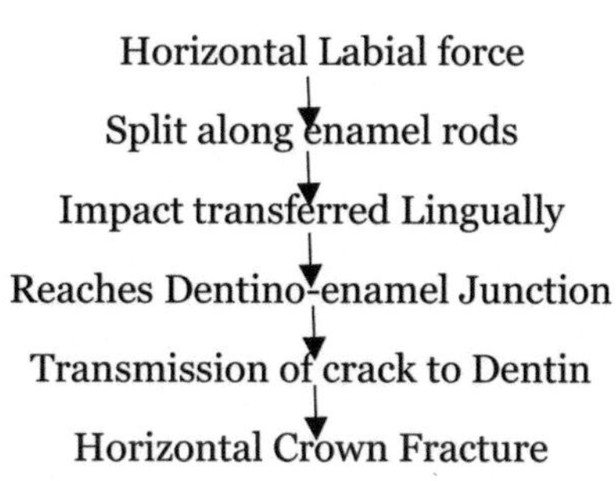

Figure 2.
Process of horizontal crown fracture.

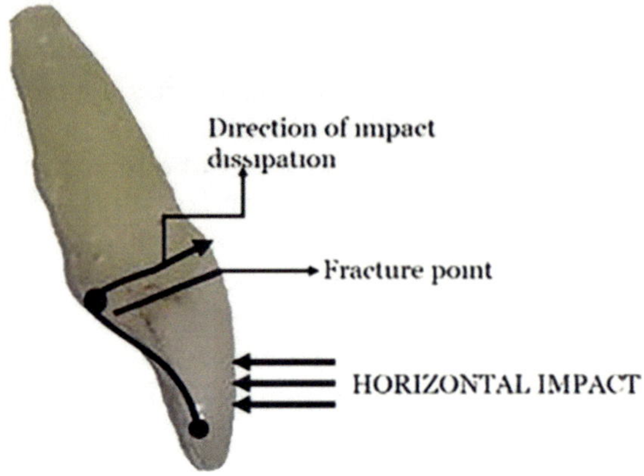

Figure 3.
Fracture point in horizontal impact.

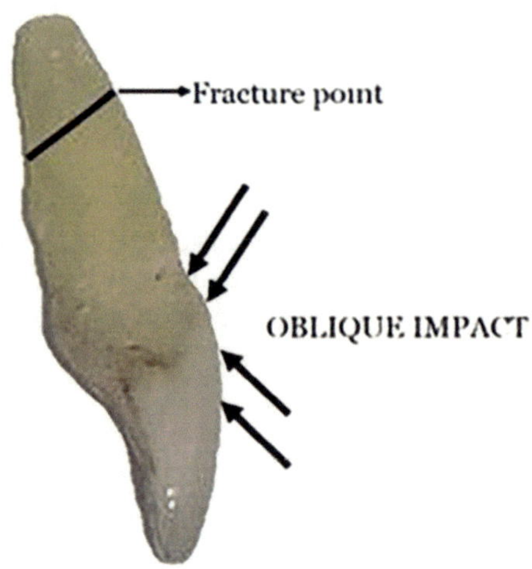

Figure 4.
Oblique impact and apical fracture point.

During such impacts, if the tooth is firmly locked in the socket, the stresses will concentrate lingually at the cervical margin and labially at the apical portion of the root. Consequently, the lines connecting these high-stress areas can lead to oblique root fractures or crown-root fractures of the tooth [4].

When a tooth encounters a vertical impact, the forces are primarily concentrated at the impact site and then progress toward the labial cervical crown. This often results in enamel crack lines by damaging the intact enamel rods (**Figure 5**).

4.2 Internal occlusal forces

The periodontal ligament cushions the impact on the crown due to its elastic properties, accommodating forces applied to the teeth [15]. As occlusal forces increase, the periodontium responds by widening the periodontal ligament space, increasing the number and width of periodontal ligament fibers, and enhancing the density of the alveolar bone. Over time, occlusal trauma can lead to adaptive tooth mobility (**Figure 6**).

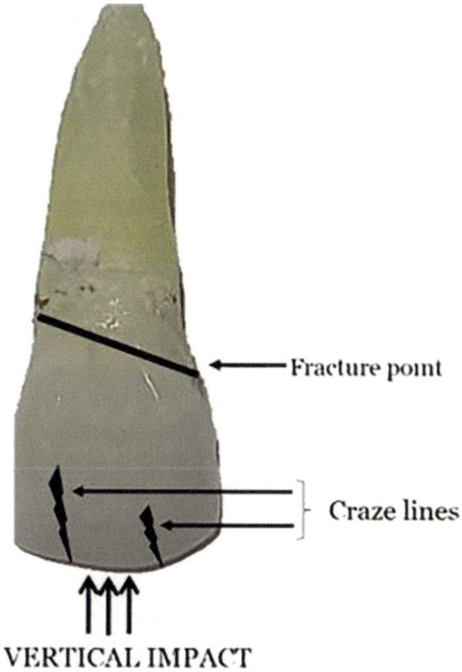

Figure 5.
Vertical impact with craze line and fracture point.

Occlusal trauma
↓
Periodontal vascular changes
↓
Stasis and Vasodilation
↓
Disruption of blood vessels walls
↓
Release of content in surrounding tissues
↓
Pain & Hypersensitivity
↓
Bone loss
↓
Periodontal ligament widening
↓
Tooth mobility

Figure 6.
Flowchart showing sequalae of occlusal trauma.

5. Response of periodontium to trauma

A healthy periodontium offers the essential support needed for functional teeth. It includes the gingival complex, periodontal ligament fibers, cementum, and alveolar bone. The proper functioning of teeth relies on the coordinated effort of these supporting structures [20].

5.1 Gingiva

The gingiva is a component of the masticatory mucosa that covers the alveolar process and encircles the cervical portions of the teeth [21]. It consists of gingival fibers made of collagen. These fibers brace the marginal gingiva firmly against the tooth and provide rigidity to withstand masticatory forces [20].

Reaction to trauma-Gingival tissues often experience trauma in the form of laceration, abrasion, and contusion. During luxation injuries, the gingival attachment is frequently torn. When trauma is limited to the gingival fiber attachment alone, healing is generally rapid and effective due to the rich blood supply to the gingival fibers. Experimental studies show that healing of traumatic gingival damage begins within a day and typically completes within 7 days, with junctional epithelium recovery and the rejoining of ruptured gingival and transseptal collagen fibers occurring after about 1 week [4].

However, if a tooth fracture occurs below the gingival margin, such as in crown-root fractures, bacterial plaque accumulation at the fracture site can lead to apical migration of the junctional epithelium, resulting in gingival recession [7].

5.2 Periodontal ligament

The periodontal ligament is a complex, highly vascularized, and cellular connective tissue that encircles the tooth root and attaches it to the inner wall of the alveolar bone. It is continuous with the connective tissue of the gingiva and communicates with the marrow spaces via vascular channels within the bone [20]. When functional demands change, the PDL adapts by adjusting the orientation, quantity, and insertion pattern of its principal fibers [4].

Reaction to trauma-The periodontal ligament can withstand forces up to approximately 16 MPa; forces beyond this threshold can cause the fibers to tear. Injuries to the periodontal tissues include concussion, subluxation, extrusive luxation, lateral luxation, intrusive luxation, and avulsion. In response to these injuries, the PDL must manage various types of stresses, including compressive, tensile, or shearing forces, which can lead to hemorrhage, edema, and rupture or contusion of the PDL.

Bleeding or edema in the PDL following minor trauma can increase pressure, potentially causing minor damage to the root surfaces. In cases of subluxation, where the impact is sufficient to loosen the tooth, this pressure may be alleviated. However, if no loosening occurs, as in concussion injuries, the increased pressure may lead to subsequent surface resorption.

When large areas (>4 mm^2) of the PDL are traumatized, competitive wound healing processes occur between bone marrow-derived stem cells, which are destined to form bone, and PDL-derived cells, which are programmed to form PDL fibers and cementum. This competition often results in ankylosis or replacement resorption. Once ankylosis sets in, it is generally permanent due to the insufficient number of surviving PDL cells relative to the extent of the damage. In contrast, if the defects are smaller than 4 mm^2, ankylosis may be transient, with potential for complete healing [4].

5.3 Cementum

Cementum is a calcified, avascular mesenchymal tissue that covers the outer surface of the anatomic root. Sharpey fibers predominantly constitute the structure of cementum, which plays a crucial role in supporting the tooth [20].

DOI: http://dx.doi.org/10.5772/intechopen.1006978

Reaction to trauma-Following root fracture, loss of cementum triggers the formation of new cementum on the exposed root dentin. This repair process begins with the activation of existing cementoblasts near the area of tissue loss. The newly formed cementum may present a multi-layered appearance similar to alveolar bone, a characteristic often resulting from transient ankylosis [4].

When the cementum layer covering the root dentin remains intact, the root may remain ankylosed without undergoing replacement resorption. However, if the cementum layer is extensively damaged along with loss of the PDL, the ankylosed root becomes integrated into the alveolar bone remodeling system. In such cases, it is gradually resorbed and replaced by bone through a process known as replacement resorption, which is influenced by the turnover rate of the bone.

5.4 Alveolar bone

The alveolar process is the part of the maxilla and mandible that forms and supports the tooth sockets (alveoli). It develops as the tooth erupts to provide osseous attachment to the periodontal ligament and gradually resorbs after tooth loss. Bone remodeling is a key process for altering bone shape, enhancing resistance to forces, repairing injuries, and maintaining calcium and phosphate balance in the body. The coupling of bone resorption and bone formation is a fundamental principle of continuous bone remodeling throughout life.

Reaction to trauma-The alveolar process can be injured through both indirect trauma, such as lateral luxation, intrusion, and avulsion, and direct trauma, such as alveolar and bone fractures. This injury triggers an inflammatory response, leading to the release of cytokines that activate osteoclasts to resorb damaged bone tissue before healing can occur [7]. The integrity of the cementoblast and odontoblast layers, which cover the cementum and dentin, respectively, is crucial. If trauma results in irreparable damage to these cell layers, the hard tissue surface may undergo resorption due to the heightened osteoclastic activity caused by osteoclast-activating factors [4].

When trauma leads to significant loss of the alveolar crest, it rarely returns to its original position. This is likely because the periodontal ligament is replaced by connective tissue from the oral mucosa, which lacks the osteogenic potential of the original PDL, resulting in loss of the crestal bone [7].

All the supporting structures of the teeth generally have good regenerative and healing potential for minor dental injuries. However, when damage exceeds the capacity for natural healing, it can result in significant adverse outcomes, leading to a compromised state of the dentition.

5.5 Response of periodontium to trauma from occlusion

When the periodontium is subjected to trauma from occlusion, healing occurs in three stages: injury, repair, and adaptive remodeling. Excessive occlusal forces cause initial tissue injury. If these forces are reduced through occlusal adjustment or natural tooth drift, the periodontium initiates its natural repair mechanisms, a process known as buttressing bone formation. If the excessive forces persist chronically, the periodontium undergoes remodeling to mitigate the impact. This results in the widening of the periodontal ligament at the expense of the surrounding bone, the development of angular bone defects without the formation of periodontal pockets, and eventual tooth mobility.

6. Trauma response of diseased periodontium

According to the 2018 World Workshop by the European Federation of Periodontology and the American Academy of Periodontology, periodontal health is defined as the absence of clinically detectable inflammation. A healthy periodontium comprises specialized tissues that support the tooth against both intraoral and extraoral forces. The previous section detailed the response of clinically healthy periodontal structures to trauma. It is an established fact that such structures possess the fight response. In contrast, individuals with pre-existing periodontal disease will exhibit a compromised healing response when subjected to traumatic dental injuries. Such diseased tissues do not respond as effectively to trauma, leading to potentially poorer healing outcomes.

Periodontitis is a disease affecting the tooth's supporting structures, including the gingival tissue, alveolar bone, cementum, and periodontal ligament. The condition is initiated and exacerbated by commensal oral bacteria through a process known as dysbiosis or microbial imbalance. Neutrophils attempt to combat the bacteria by engulfing them, but when they become overwhelmed, they rupture, releasing toxins and enzymes that irritate the periodontal tissues and cause inflammation of the gingival margin. This inflammation results in the loosening of the attached gingiva from the tooth, creating a periodontal pocket. As periodontitis progresses, it leads to the detachment of periodontal ligament fibers and a weakening of the tooth's support system, eventually causing alveolar bone loss. This loss of bone reduces tooth anchorage and strength. Additionally, affected teeth may experience pathological migration, especially in the anterior region, leading to proclination, flaring, and supraeruption. These changes increase the susceptibility of the teeth to traumatic injury.

There is evidence suggesting that bacteria-induced gingival inflammation can adversely affect wound healing following trauma [4]. If an odontogenic infection from a tooth fracture extends from the bone marrow to the periosteal layer, leading to an abscess formation between the periosteum and cortical bone, the blood supply to the underlying cortical bone may be compromised. This can result in ischemic necrosis of the cortical bone, leading to undermining resorption [22]. Consequently, this further weakens the overall support system of the tooth, making it more susceptible to additional damage.

Periodontally compromised teeth are generally weaker than healthy teeth due to the loss of natural support and ongoing infection. When such teeth are subjected to trauma, the center of resistance shifts, causing the tooth to deflect more and increasing the risk of complete avulsion. Additionally, soft tissue lacerations are more frequent and severe in these cases due to existing inflammation and tissue fragility. Minor traumatic injuries can exacerbate into more severe conditions, especially in younger individuals who are more prone to traumatic dental injuries and often having inadequate oral hygiene can increase the likelihood of tooth loss from seemingly minor trauma.

This highlights the need for raising awareness about dental trauma, emphasizing the importance of regular dental check-ups and consistent oral hygiene maintenance. By motivating patients to adhere to these practices, potential issues can be addressed promptly and effectively, minimizing the risk of serious complications.

7. Management and periodontal protection

The initial post-trauma visit is crucial for assessing the extent of the injury and determining the most effective treatment approach. The long-term prognosis of traumatized teeth significantly relies on timely and appropriate emergency care [23].

The following outlines some of the management protocols to be followed when treating a patient with a traumatic dental injury.

First, a detailed history of the incident should be obtained. During history taking, important questions to ask include: "When did the injury occur? How did it happen? Where did it take place? What immediate care was administered? Was there any loss of consciousness? Is there any previous history of similar trauma?" and so on. A comprehensive assessment is crucial for developing a diagnosis and treatment plan that ensures a favorable and lasting outcome. To guide the initial assessment, remember the mnemonic *HEST* (History, Examination, and Special Test).

The extraoral examination should focus on identifying swelling, lacerations, abrasions, bruises, and soft tissue loss, remembered with the mnemonic *SLABS*. Special attention should be given to severe bruising around the eyes, checking for any deformity of the infraorbital rim. For significant tissue lacerations and open wounds, suturing should be performed. If a fractured mandible or facial fracture is suspected based on the impact and forces involved, the lower mandible should be examined, and the patient should be urgently referred to a maxillofacial unit [24].

The intraoral examination involves assessing both soft and hard tissues.

7.1 Soft tissue trauma

7.1.1 Gingiva

Minor bruising of the gingiva may result in mild bleeding from the gingival margin, indicating a tear in the gingival fibers. This bleeding can generally be controlled with measures to stop it. In cases of severe gingival inflammation due to local factors, gross scaling under local anesthesia may be necessary to halt the bleeding. Patients should be placed on a plaque control regimen with ongoing monitoring. If trauma causes deep gingival injury and significant bleeding, indicating a tear in the periodontal ligament fibers, periodontal management and stabilization of the affected teeth are required. The process of stabilizing teeth will be discussed further.

7.1.2 Buccal or labial mucosa

Severe lacerations of the mucosa can result in intense pain and bleeding. The lower labial mucosa is often affected by fragments of broken teeth following trauma. In such instances, the foreign object or broken tooth fragment should be removed immediately under anesthesia, with a blunt incision and sutures as needed. Pain management and, if necessary, antibiotic therapy should also be provided.

7.2 Hard tissue trauma

7.2.1 Alveolar bone

Digital palpation should be employed to check for any step formation within the alveolar bone, which may indicate a fracture. If a fracture is detected, follow the fracture management protocol and refer the patient to an oral and maxillofacial specialist for further care. The treatment typically involves repositioning any displaced segments and applying a splint. The affected segment should be stabilized for approximately 4 weeks.

7.2.2 Teeth

There are different parts of teeth that can be involved in the trauma. The management of traumatic dental injuries often requires a multidisciplinary approach involving endodontics, orthodontics, periodontics, implantology, prosthodontics, and oral surgery. Following **Table 3** gives a brief view of management protocol stated by the International Academy of Dental Traumatology (IADT) [25].

Trauma	Treatment
1. Infraction	• For significant infractions, resin etching and sealing can prevent discoloration along the cracks.
2. Enamel fracture	• If the tooth fragment is available, it can be bonded back to the tooth. Alternatively, contouring or restoration with composite resin may be used, depending on the extent and location of the fracture.
3. Enamel-dentin fracture:	• If the tooth fragment is available, it can be bonded back to the tooth. If not, provide provisional treatment by covering the exposed dentin with glass ionomer, or apply a more permanent restoration using a bonding agent and composite resin. • If the exposed dentin is within 0.5 mm of the pulp, place a calcium hydroxide base and cover it with a material such as glass ionomer.
4. Enamel-dentin-pulp fracture	• For young patients with immature, developing teeth, pulp capping or a partial pulpotomy can be considered. • For patients with mature apical development, root canal treatment is typically the preferred option.
5. Crown-root fracture without pulp exposure:	*Emergency treatment*: Temporarily stabilize the loose segment to adjacent teeth until a definitive treatment plan can be determined. *Non-emergency treatment alternatives*: • Fragment removal only. • Fragment removal followed by endodontic treatment and restoration with a post-retained crown. • Orthodontic extrusion of apical fragment • Surgical extrusion to reposition the root to a more coronal position. • Root submergence • Extraction: Extract the tooth and consider immediate or delayed restoration.
6. Crown-root fracture with pulp exposure	*Emergency Treatment*: Temporarily stabilize the loose segment to adjacent teeth. In patients with open apices, partial pulpotomy is beneficial. For patients with mature apices, root canal treatment is typically preferred. *Non-emergency treatment alternatives*: Follow the same protocol as for crown-root fractures without pulp exposure.
7. Root fracture	If the coronal segment is displaced, reposition it as soon as possible. Verify the position radiographically. Stabilize the tooth with a flexible splint for 4 weeks. If the fracture is near the cervical area, extend stabilization up to 4 months for better results. Monitor the healing process for at least one year to assess the pulpal status. If pulp necrosis occurs, perform root canal treatment.
8. Concussion	No specific treatment is required. Observe the pulpal condition for at least one year to ensure no delayed complications arise.
9. Subluxation	Typically, no specific treatment is required. However, a flexible splint can be used to stabilize the tooth and provide patient comfort for up to 2 weeks.
10. Extrusive luxation	Gently reinsert the tooth into its socket. Use a flexible splint to stabilize the tooth for 2 weeks. If pulp necrosis is expected, root canal treatment is necessary.

Trauma	Treatment
11. Lateral luxation	Use digital manipulation or forceps to disengage the tooth from its bony lock and gently reposition it into its original location. Stabilize the tooth with a flexible splint for 4 weeks. Regularly monitor the pulpal condition. If the pulp becomes necrotic, root canal treatment is required to prevent root resorption.
12. Intrusive luxation	*Teeth with incomplete root formation:* • Allow the tooth to erupt naturally without intervention. If there is no movement within a few weeks, consider initiating orthodontic repositioning. For intrusions greater than 7 mm, surgical or orthodontic repositioning is necessary. *Teeth with complete root formation:* • If the tooth is intruded less than 3 mm, allow natural eruption. If no movement is observed after 2–4 weeks, reposition surgically or orthodontically to prevent ankylosis. • For intrusions of 3–7 mm, reposition the tooth either surgically or orthodontically. • If the intrusion exceeds 7 mm, surgical repositioning is required. • Pulp necrosis is likely in teeth with complete root formation. Root canal therapy should begin 2–3 weeks after repositioning. • After surgical or orthodontic repositioning, stabilize the tooth with a flexible splint for 4 weeks.

Table 3.
Brief overview of IADT guidelines.

7.3 Avulsion

Management:

- Treatment choice depends on the root's maturity (whether it has an open or closed apex) and the health of the periodontal ligament cells.

Condition of periodontal ligament cells:

- Immediate reimplantation: PDL cells are most likely to be viable.
- Short-term storage: If the tooth was stored in a suitable medium (e.g., tissue culture medium, HBSS, saline, milk, or saliva) and the total extraoral dry time is less than 60 minutes, the PDL cells may be viable but possibly compromised.
- Extended dry time: If the tooth has been out of the mouth for more than 60 minutes, regardless of storage medium, the PDL cells are likely non-viable.

Line of treatment for avulsed permanent teeth with closed apex

a. If the tooth is replanted before arriving at the clinic:

   - Keep the tooth in place. Rinse the area thoroughly with saline or chlorhexidine solution. Suture any gingival lacerations as needed. Check the tooth's position both clinically and radiographically. Apply a splint to stabilize the tooth for 2 weeks. Schedule follow-ups, prescribe medications if necessary, and perform root canal treatment at least a week after replantation before removing the splint.

b. If the tooth is carried in a viable storage medium within an hour of the accident:

- Assess the tooth for secondary trauma and clean it thoroughly to remove debris. Ensure adequate anesthesia, then clean and irrigate the socket. Replant the tooth and confirm its position with a radiograph. Apply a splint for 2 weeks, prescribe medications if needed, and suture any gingival lacerations. Perform root canal treatment 7–10 days after replantation before removing the splint.

c. If the tooth's extraoral dry time is more than an hour:

- Attempt delayed replantation. Clean the tooth properly with saline. Under aseptic conditions, perform root canal treatment. Replant the tooth into the socket under anesthesia after copious irrigation of the socket. Follow the same steps as mentioned above for splinting and regular follow-ups, but plan to remove the splint only after 4 weeks.

Line of treatment for avulsed permanent teeth with open apex

a. Immediate replantation of the tooth:

- Protocol: Follow the same protocol as for closed apex teeth.

b. Within 1 hour of trauma:

- Replant the tooth if it was stored in an appropriate medium after thorough cleaning. Applying topical antibiotics to the tooth surface may enhance revascularization.

- Protocol: Follow the same protocol as for closed apex teeth.

c. Extraoral time more than 1 hour:

- Protocol: Follow the same protocol as for closed apex teeth.

7.4 Periodontal splint: A means of periodontal protection

Definition: According to the 2001 Glossary of Periodontal Terms, a splint is an appliance designed to immobilize and stabilize loose teeth. A periodontal splint is specifically used to maintain, stabilize, or immobilize mobile teeth in their functional and physiological positions [26].

Current recommendations: [27].

- Type of splint: Use passive and flexible splints.

- Duration: Employ for a short-term period.

- Application: Suitable for splinting teeth that have been avulsed, luxated, or root-fractured.

Material type	Examples
RESINS	Composite resins, e.g., bonded splints; acrylic resins, e.g., night guards.
WIRE	Braided wires, soft stainless steel wire (<0.3–0.4 mm diameter).
BRIDGES	Maryland bridges, Conevtional bridges.
RIBBONS/STRIPS	Resin-reinforced ribbons/strips; fiber-reinforced composite splints.

Table 4.
Materials used for splinting.

Purpose: The primary goal of a periodontal splint is to stabilize the affected teeth and aid in their recovery by keeping them in their proper positions.

Periodontal splints are available in various materials (**Table 4**) and serve the fundamental purpose of stabilizing the tooth and distributing forces evenly. Their primary functions include reducing the burden on individual teeth and enhancing the potential for attachment gain. A stable tooth is more likely to achieve attachment gain compared to a mobile one.

Key characteristics:

- Flexibility: The splint should ideally have slight vertical and horizontal flexibility. This flexibility supports the healing process by accommodating natural tooth movement and maintaining the repositioned tooth.

- Function: Properly designed splints improve function and support the healing of the affected tooth.

Incorporating these features into the splint design ensures optimal stabilization and healing outcomes for traumatized teeth.

Rigidity of splints

a. Flexible splint: It allows more mobility than a non-injured tooth. Commonly used for traumatized teeth to accommodate natural tooth movement and facilitate recovery of the periodontium and reorganization of periodontal ligament fibers.

b. Semi-rigid splint: It provides mobility equivalent to a normal tooth. Promote collagen production and maturation through fibril polymerization, enhancing the recovery of the periodontal ligament.

c. Rigid splints: It allows less movement than a normal tooth. Its extended use may lead to ankylosis and external replacement resorption due to the lack of movement [28].

Precaution during splinting:

Keep composite and bonding agents away from gingival margins and proximal areas to prevent plaque buildup, secondary caries, or infection.

8. Digitization and artificial intelligence in dental trauma

Digital dentistry has made its way into nearly every aspect of dental practice. Adequate stabilization of the tooth is key to periodontal healing. Digitally printed splints used often offer improved adaptability to teeth and enhanced stabilization. A study by Churen et al. indicates the effectiveness of using 3D-printed periodontal splints [29].

Clinical practice shows that a more comprehensive examination leads to more effective treatment. A practical application of artificial intelligence (AI) is through knowledge-based systems (KBS), which offer substantial support to caregivers. With the assistance of AI, a well-known program like XpertRule (Attar, London) can analyze input data to predict dental injuries in children. This information can then be used to help prevent dental trauma [30]. AI can also be utilized in database collection and management. It helps create detailed treatment plans for specific types of traumatic dental injuries, resulting in more accurate judgments and improved treatment outcomes.

9. Conclusion

Dental trauma is not a new concept in dentistry; however, managing such cases remains consistently challenging. Dentists require specialized training to accurately identify the type of injury, understand its causes and related factors, manage the trauma effectively, and motivate the patient. Dental trauma should be included in first aid guideline books for medical and non-medical professionals, as these are unavoidable situations. Staying updated and informed can help reduce the risk of long-term damage.

Acknowledgements

I would like to extend my heartfelt gratitude to those who contributed to the development and completion of this chapter, in particular, Dr. A V Ramesh, whose guidance and insightful feedback were invaluable throughout this process and my guru, and Dr. Lalith Vivekananda for a constant source of motivation, support, and unwavering belief in me. I also want to acknowledge the support of the Dental Health Clinic team, which provided the resources and environment necessary for the completion of this chapter. Lastly, my sincere thanks go to my family and friends for their patience and understanding during the demanding writing process. Thank you all for your contributions and encouragement.

Conflict of interest

None declared.

Nomenclature

TDI	Traumatic dental injury
PDL	periodontal ligament
DEJ	Dentino-enamel junction
FEA	Finite Element Analysis
AI	Artificial Intelligence

DOI: http://dx.doi.org/10.5772/intechopen.1006978

Author details

Kumari Abhilasha
Private Practitioner, Quad Care Dental and Derma, Bengaluru, Karnataka, India

*Address all correspondence to: drk.abhilasha@gmail.com

References

[1] Bezroukov V. The application of the international classification of diseases to dentistry and stomatology. Community Dentistry and Oral Epidemiology. 1979;**7**(1):21-24

[2] Pagadala S, Tadikonda DC. An overview of classification of dental trauma. International Archives of Integrated Medicine. 2015;**2**(9):157-164

[3] Zaleckiene V, Peciuliene V, Brukiene V, Drukteinis S. Traumatic dental injuries: Etiology, prevalence and possible outcomes. Stomatologija. 2014;**16**(1):7-14

[4] Andreasen JO, Andreasen FM, Andersson L. Textbook and Color Atlas of Traumatic Injuries to the Teeth. United Kingdom: John Wiley and Sons; 2018

[5] Judd MA, Redfern R. Trauma. In: Grauer AL, editor. Encyclopedia of Paleopathology. Oxford: Blackwells Wiley-Liss; 2012. pp. 359-379

[6] Mordini L, Lee P, Lazaro R, Biagi R, Giannetti L. Sport and dental traumatology: Surgical solutions and prevention. Dentistry Journal. 2021;**9**(3):33

[7] Yu CY, Abbott PV. Responses of the pulp, periradicular and soft tissues following trauma to the permanent teeth. Australian Dental Journal. 2016;**61**:39-58

[8] Oikarinen K. Pathogenesis and mechanism of traumatic injuries to teeth. Dental Traumatology. 1987;**3**(5):220-223

[9] Jayasudha K, Hemanth M, Baswa R, Raghuveer HP, Vedavathi B, Hegde C. Traumatic impact loading on human maxillary incisor: A dynamic finite element analysis. Journal of Indian Society of Pedodontics and Preventive Dentistry. 2015;**33**(4):302-306

[10] Caeiro-Villasenin L, Serna-Munoz C, Perez-Silva A, Vicente-Hernandez A, Poza-Pascual A, Ortiz-Ruiz AJ. Developmental dental defects in permanent teeth resulting from trauma in primary dentition: A systematic review. International Journal of Environmental Research and Public Health. 2022;**19**(2):754

[11] Özükoç C, Kanat A. Evaluation of the traumatic dental injuries in mixed dentition. Evaluation. 2019;**5**(9):9-12

[12] Andreasen JO, Bakland LK, Andreasen FM. Traumatic intrusion of permanent teeth. Part 2. A clinical study of the effect of preinjury and injury factors, such as sex, age, stage of root development, tooth location, and extent of injury including number of intruded teeth on 140 intruded permanent teeth. Dental Traumatology. 2006;**22**:90-98

[13] Hermann NV, Lauridsen E, Ahrensburg SS, Gerds TA, Andreasen JO. Periodontal healing complications following extrusive and lateral luxation in the permanent dentition: A longitudinal cohort study. Dental Traumatology. 2012;**28**:394-402

[14] de Andrade Veras SR, Bem JS, de Almeida EC, Lins CC. Dental splints: Types and time of immobilization post tooth avulsion. Journal of Istanbul University Faculty of Dentistry. 2017;**51**(3 Suppl_1):S69

[15] Mahendra J, AbiramiNayaki Rao P, Janani M. Trauma from occlusion-periodontal traumatism. Annals of the Romanian Society for Cell Biology. 2020;**24**(1):1224-1236

[16] Biancu S, Ericsson I, Lindhe J. Periodontal ligament tissue reactions to trauma and gingival inflammation: An experimental study in the beagle dog. Journal of Clinical Periodontology. 1995;**22**(10):772-779

[17] Hughes CE, White CA. Crack propagation in teeth: A comparison of perimortem and postmortem behavior of dental materials and cracks. Journal of Forensic Sciences. 2009;**54**(2):263-266

[18] Imbeni V, Kruzic JJ, Marshall GW, Marshall SJ, Ritchie RO. The dentin–enamel junction and the fracture of human teeth. Nature Materials. 2005;**4**(3):229-232

[19] Al-Mukhtar AM. Fracture mechanism in human teeth. Procedia Structural Integrity. 2020;**25**:8-12

[20] Newman MG, Takei H, Klokkevold PR, Carranza FA. Newman and Carranza's Clinical Periodontology. United States: Elsevier Health Sciences; 2018

[21] Lindhe J, Karring T, Lang NP. Clinical Periodontology and Implant Dentistry. United Kingdom: Blackwell; 2003

[22] Yamasaki A, Rose GG, Pinero GJ, Manan CJ. Ultrastructural and morphometric analyses of human cementoblasts and periodontal fibroblasts. Journal of Periodontology. 1987;**58**(3):192-201

[23] Hinckfuss SE, Messer LB. Splinting duration and periodontal outcomes for replanted avulsed teeth: A systematic review. Dental Traumatology. 2009;**25**(2):150-157

[24] Djemal S. Dental Trauma: A Practical Guide to Diagnosis and Management. India: JP Medical Ltd; 2021

[25] Traumatology D. International association of dental traumatology. Dental Trauma Guidelines Revised 2012. United States: Iadt; 2012

[26] Bhuvaneswari P, Gowri T, Kumar R, Vanitha M. Periodontal splinting: A review before planning a splint. International Journal of Applied Dental Sciences. 2019;**5**(4):315-319

[27] Mehrabi F, Djemal S. International association for dental traumatology guideline updates. British Dental Journal. 2021;**230**(10):671-675

[28] Gupta R, Tomer AK, Parvathi Jayan S. Recent advances in splinting in dentistry. IOSR Journal of Dental and Medical Sciences (IOSR-JDMS). 2023;**22**(06):37-43

[29] Zhang C, Liu Q, Yang J, Hou J. A digital technique for splinting periodontally compromised mobile teeth in the mandibular anterior region. The Journal of Prosthetic Dentistry. 2021;**125**(4):560-563

[30] Shaikh K, Bekal SV, Marei HF, Elsayed WS, Surdilovic D, Jawad LA. Artificial Intelligence in Dentistry. Germany: Springer Nature; 2022

Chapter 4

Association between Dental Trauma and Periodontal Disease

Elena Furman

Abstract

This chapter aims to explore the link between dental trauma and the development and progression of periodontal disease. It reviews the epidemiology, classification, and signs and symptoms of periodontal disease, noting its widespread prevalence and key risk factors. Further, it emphasizes the role of inflammatory response to bacterial plaque and trauma-induced changes in periodontium. The chapter addresses different forms of trauma, including occlusal trauma, dental trauma associated with physical injuries, and psychological trauma. While the mechanical impact of occlusal trauma or traumatic dental injury can impair the tooth's support system, psychological trauma, as a stress factor, is also considered for its indirect effect on periodontal health. Mechanisms linking trauma and periodontal disease include biomechanical stress, inflammatory pathways, and immune system dysregulation. The chapter provides an integrated view of how dental, occlusal, or psychological trauma can contribute to the onset or worsening of periodontal disease using current scientific evidence. Treatment strategies focus on prevention, early intervention, appropriate management of traumatic injuries, and long-term periodontal maintenance. Clinical recommendations highlight the importance of multidisciplinary care, including comprehensive assessment, collaboration with mental health professionals, and an emphasis on the importance of maintaining good oral hygiene. This chapter advocates for timely treatment and long-term monitoring of trauma-affected patients to prevent or manage periodontal complications.

Keywords: periodontal disease, trauma, occlusal trauma, physical trauma, physiological trauma

1. Introduction

Dental trauma and periodontal disease are conditions that may affect someone's health and well-being. While very different in origin, these two conditions are interconnected through complex relationships involving both direct injury and secondary effects on the periodontal tissues. Trauma to the teeth, whether through accidents or occlusal dysfunction, can exacerbate or trigger periodontal problems, while existing periodontal disease can influence the severity of dental injuries. Additionally, patients experiencing these conditions often present with dental anxiety, which further complicates diagnosis and treatment. This chapter explores the interlaced and multilayered relationships between dental trauma, occlusal trauma, and periodontal disease, while also addressing the role of dental anxiety in the management of these conditions. Based on the available data from PubMed, Google Scholar, and Web of Science database, this chapter will outline the latest information available on this topic, including epidemiology, classification, diagnosis, and treatment strategies.

2. Periodontal disease

According to the American Academy of Periodontology, periodontal disease encompasses a group of infectious and inflammatory diseases that affect the tissues that surround and support teeth. These tissues include gingiva, cementum, periodontal ligament, and alveolar bone, collectively called periodontium [1]. The primary forms of periodontal disease are gingivitis and periodontitis. Gingivitis is an inflammation limited to the gingiva without attachment loss, while periodontitis involves loss of periodontal attachment and destruction of alveolar bone.

2.1 Epidemiology

Periodontal disease is highly prevalent worldwide. According to the Global Burden of Disease Study, approximately 45% of adults over the age of 30 suffer from periodontitis, with severe cases affecting around 10% of the global adult population [2]. According to data from the National Health and Nutrition Examination Survey 2009–2014, 42% of adults in the United States had periodontitis, with 7.8% having severe periodontitis [3].

The prevalence increases with age, and socioeconomic factors such as lower income and education levels are associated with higher incidence rates. In the U.S., the National Institute of Dental and Craniofacial Research (NIDCR) estimates that nearly 70% of adults aged 65 and older have periodontitis. Other factors influencing periodontal disease prevalence include smoking, diabetes, and genetic predispositions [4]. Although Periodontal disease is traditionally associated with adults, an increasing body of evidence shows that "gum disease" can also affect children and adolescents, albeit with some distinctions in its etiology, progression, and clinical presentation. Recent updates in the classification of periodontal diseases emphasize the need to recognize and address periodontitis in younger populations to prevent long-term consequences. Periodontitis in children and adolescents differs from that in adults in terms of its underlying causes, disease progression, and response to treatment. While the prevalence of periodontitis is lower in younger populations, the disease can have severe implications if left untreated. Periodontitis is relatively rare in children, with more cases seen in adolescents and young adults. Data suggests that aggressive forms of periodontitis may affect 0.1% to 0.5% of adolescents worldwide, with some regional variations. Localized aggressive periodontitis (LAP) tends to manifest during puberty, while generalized aggressive periodontitis (GAP) can present later, usually during the late teenage years or early twenties. The Global Burden of Disease Study emphasizes the significant impact of severe periodontal disease on quality of life, even in younger populations, underscoring the need for early detection and management.

2.2 Classification

The American Academy of Periodontology (AAP) updated its classification system in 2017 to provide a clearer framework for diagnosing and managing periodontal diseases [5]. The classification system divides periodontal diseases into several categories:

1. Gingival diseases

    a. *Gingivitis:* Inflammation of the gingiva without loss of attachment or bone.

    b. *Systemic conditions affecting the gingiva:* Including conditions such as pregnancy or medication-induced gingival overgrowth.

2. Periodontitis

    a. *Necrotizing periodontal diseases:* Includes necrotizing ulcerative gingivitis (NUG) and necrotizing ulcerative periodontitis (NUP).

    b. *Periodontitis:* Classified into:

        i. *Periodontitis Stage I (Initial):* Characterized by initial attachment loss.

        ii. *Periodontitis Stage II (Moderate):* Moderate attachment loss with increased complexity.

        iii. *Periodontitis Stage III (Severe with Potential for Additional Tooth Loss):* Severe attachment loss and significant clinical complexity.

        iv. *Periodontitis Stage IV (Advanced with Potential for Loss of Dentition):* Advanced attachment loss with extensive tooth mobility or loss.

3. Each stage is further classified by:

    a. *Extent and distribution:* Localized (less than 30% of teeth affected) or generalized (more than 30% of teeth affected).

    b. *Complexity of management:* Based on the severity and complexity of the disease, which affects treatment planning.

4. *Other conditions:*

    a. *Periodontal manifestations of systemic diseases:* Including genetic disorders or systemic conditions that affect periodontal tissues.

    b. *Other periodontal conditions:* Such as occlusal trauma or dental abscesses.

2.3 Etiology and pathogenesis

The pathogenesis of periodontitis in younger individuals shares similarities with adult periodontitis, involving a complex interplay of microbial colonization, host immune response, and genetic predispositions. Even though the etiology of periodontal disease is multifactorial, according to systematic reviews, the primary etiology of periodontal disease is bacterial plaque/biofilm. This biofilm is composed of various bacteria that adhere to the teeth and gingival tissues, initiating an inflammatory response in the host. Over time, if the biofilm is not adequately removed, it leads to the development of gingivitis, which can progress to periodontitis in susceptible individuals. The microbial composition of the biofilm, especially the presence of pathogenic bacteria such as *Porphyromonas Gingivalis*, *Tannerella Forsythia*, and *Treponema Denticola*, plays a crucial role in the development and progression of periodontal disease. These bacteria are collectively known as the "red complex" and are associated with more severe forms of periodontitis [6]. While microbial plaque is the initiating factor, the host's immune response significantly determines the severity and progression of periodontal disease. An exaggerated or dysregulated immune response to bacterial invasion can result in the destruction of the periodontal ligament and alveolar bone, leading to tooth mobility and loss [7].

2.4 Clinical signs and symptoms

Clinically gingivitis is manifested by redness and edema in the gingiva without clinical attachment loss. Primary clinical signs and symptoms of gingivitis include swollen and tender gums that may bleed easily during brushing and flossing. Gingivitis is often associated with poor oral hygiene, leading to plaque and calculus buildup along the gingival line. Gingivitis is usually painless, however, it can be associated with ulcers and pain in the case of Acute Ulcerative Gingivitis. With proper oral care and treatment, gingivitis can be reversed before it progresses to periodontitis when damage to the bone and supporting tissues is irreversible.

Periodontitis is characterized by clinical attachment loss (loss of the periodontal tissue support) and formation of the periodontal pockets due to distraction of the periodontal ligament and alveolar bone. In advanced cases, it may lead to increased tooth mobility or tooth loss. Patients may complain of pain when eating, brushing, or flossing. Patients may experience persistent bad breath (halitosis), gum recession that makes teeth appear longer. As a result of reduced periodontal support, teeth may shift, creating changes in occlusion and aesthetics.

3. Occlusal trauma and its role in periodontal disease

The relationship between occlusal trauma and periodontitis has been studied for years. According to the Glossary of Periodontal Terms (American Academy of Periodontology), occlusal trauma is an injury resulting in tissue changes within the attachment apparatus due to physiologic or parafunctional forces that may exceed its adaptive capacity. These changes can occur in the periodontal ligament, cementum, and supporting alveolar bone leading to adaptive mobility of the teeth, root resorption, and tooth fracture, It can be caused by preliminary contact, parafunctions (clenching of teeth, bruxism) or migration of teeth due to tooth loss. Synonyms of occlusal trauma used in practice are also: traumatic occlusion, periodontal trauma, traumatogenic occlusion, trauma of occlusion, etc. [8]. The changes that occur in the periodontal tissues depend on the strength, direction, duration, and frequency of increased traumatic occlusal forces [9]. Occlusal trauma can be classified according to the type and duration of traumatic forces (acute and chronic) and according to the state of the periodontal tissues (primary and secondary). Acute occlusal trauma is most often caused by severe force in a short period of time: for example, biting on olive pyrene. It can be associated with acute pain, sensitivity to percussion and increased tooth mobility, fremitus, sensitivity to thermal irritation, and tooth fracture [10, 11]. Chronic occlusal trauma leads to changes in periodontal tissues associated with gradual discrepancies in occlusion due to tooth abrasion, migration, and extrusion of teeth in combination with parafunctional factors (e.g., bruxism) and non-carious cervical lesions (NCCLs) [12]. Primary occlusal trauma occurs when excessive forces are applied to teeth with healthy periodontium. While it does not directly cause periodontal disease, it can lead to increased tooth mobility and discomfort. Secondary occlusal trauma occurs when normal or excessive forces are applied to teeth with compromised periodontium, such as those affected by periodontal disease. In this case, occlusal trauma can exacerbate bone loss and mobility, accelerating the progression of periodontal disease.

Occlusal trauma can be reversed. When the excessive occlusal forces are eliminated, the tissues of the periodontium are restored [13, 14]. In cases of plaque-induced periodontal inflammation and the presence of secondary occlusal trauma, this condition is more difficult to reverse [15]. In radiographic examination, it is characterized by enlargement of the periodontal ligament space and root resorption, and possible angular bony defects.

Studies have demonstrated that occlusal trauma does not independently cause periodontal disease, but it can exacerbate the condition when periodontal tissues are already weakened. This is parand ticularly concerning in patients with untreated or poorly managed periodontal disease, where occlusal trauma can accelerate tooth loss.

4. Dental trauma associated with physical injury

Dental trauma refers to injuries to the teeth and surrounding structures, most commonly resulting from accidents, falls, sports injuries, and physical altercations. It is usually unexpected and sudden and usually requested emergency treatment. The prevalence of dental trauma is significant, with studies indicating that up to 30% of children experience some form of dental injury before adulthood. Epidemiological studies indicate the annual incidence of dental trauma globally is at about 4.5%. Approximately one-third of children and toddlers (primary teeth) and one-fifth of adolescents and adults (permanent teeth) sustained a traumatic dental injury [16]. The majority involved the maxillary central incisors, mainly from falls in toddlers at home and contact sports or accidentsin adolescents. Despite these trends, there is considerable variation between different studies. A national survey carried out in the USA, with a cohort of 154 million people between the ages of 6 and 50, revealed that almost one in three 6 to 20-year-olds and one in four 20 to 50-year-olds had suffered some form of dental traumatic injury [17].

Although these injuries are more common in certain groups of the population, no individual is ever at zero risk through their activities of daily life. These injuries may render an individual with meticulous oral hygiene and a life experience of only the standard check-up and clean with life-changing dentistry. Costs to the injured person and the community throughout the world have been substantial [18].

Dental trauma is often more time-consuming and costly compared with many other accidental injuries presented to emergency clinics and hospitals [19]. In order to recognize and treat traumatic dental injuries properly and communicate between different specialties multiple classifications were used. In fact, more than 50 different classifications exist. The commonly used one is based on a classification developed by Dr. Jens Ove Andreasen in 1970 with further modifications [20]. Based on the tissue involved, dental injuries are often classified into three categories: (Injury to the hard dental tissue, pulp, and supporting structures)

a. Enamel fracture

b. Enamel/dentin fracture

c. Complicated crown fracture

1. Injury to the hard dental tissue, pulp, and alveolar process

    a. Crown-root fracture

    b. Root fracture

    c. Alveolar fracture

2. Injury to periodontal tissue

    a. Concussion

    b. Subluxation

    c. Luxation injuries

    d. Lateral luxation

    e. Intrusion

    f. Extrusion

    g. Avulsion

While the immediate concerns following dental trauma are pain management and structural restoration, there is a growing understanding of how trauma can initiate or worsen periodontal disease. Injuries to the periodontal ligament and surrounding alveolar bone can impair the tooth's support system, leading to mobility, bone loss, and periodontal pocket formation over time.

5. Psychological trauma associated with dental injury

Traumatic dental injuries can significantly contribute to dental fear and anxiety, leading to long-term psychological trauma. Research shows that individuals who have experienced a dental injury, especially in childhood or adolescence, are at higher risk of developing dental anxiety due to acute pain, shock, and emotional distress associated with traumatic events. The sudden nature of the injury, often linked to accidents, falls, sports, or violence can imprint a lasting psychological impact, causing patients to fear dental visits or treatments. Studies indicate that up to 30% of people with dental anxiety report a previous traumatic dental injury or experience as the root cause.

It also has been shown that children with dental anxiety have poorer oral health: more severe caries, and an increased number of missing teeth [21]. Dental fear can manifest psychologically through heightened stress responses during dental visits, including increased heart rate, sweating, or panic attacks. Over time, avoidance of dental care due to fear may worsen oral health, exacerbating the cycle of anxiety and the potential for further trauma. Several studies have shown that traumatic dental injuries are associated with increased levels of anxiety and stress. For instance, a study by Eklund et al. [22] found that dental trauma could be a significant stressor leading to long-term psychological distress, including PTSD and depression. The fear of ongoing dental issues and potential alterations in appearance can exacerbate psychological strain [22]. PTSD is a mental health condition triggered by exposure to a traumatic event. Symptoms include reliving the traumatic event, avoidance of reminders, and heightened arousal. Individuals who experience traumatic dental injuries may develop PTSD due to the trauma associated with the injury and the subsequent pain and disruption in their lives.

A study by Grembowski et al. is indicated that patients with dental trauma are at a higher risk of developing PTSD symptoms. The psychological impact of such trauma can lead to increased vulnerability to PTSD, as the trauma from the dental injury can disrupt normal coping mechanisms and contribute to chronic stress [23]. Depression is commonly linked with PTSD and can be exacerbated by the stress of a traumatic dental injury. The relationship between dental trauma and depression is bidirectional, with traumatic experiences increasing the risk of depression and vice versa. Research by Mäki et al. shows that individuals with dental trauma are more likely to experience depressive symptoms, likely due to the stress and trauma of the injury and its impact on self-esteem and quality of life [24]. Psychologicalstress, including PTSD and depression, can negatively impact oral health. Chronic stress is known to affect immune function and inflammatory responses, which can exacerbate periodontal conditions. A study by Kiecolt-Glaser et al. found that psychological stress can impair the body's ability to combat periodontal disease by affecting immune response and inflammatory pathways [25].

Furthermore, individuals with PTSD and depression may exhibit poorer oral hygiene practices, which can increase the risk of periodontitis. They might avoid regular dental visits and exhibit less care in maintaining oral health, contributing to the progression of periodontal disease [26, 27].

6. Mechanism linking trauma and periodontal disease: Connecting the dots

It is known that dental trauma, even in its mildest form, invariably injuries the periodontal ligament fibers.

Dental trauma includes injuries such as fractures, avulsions, and luxations. Such trauma can disrupt normal oral function and contribute to inflammation of the gingival tissues. The immediate response to dental trauma often involves pain, swelling, and potential disruption of normal dental care routines. While the immediate concerns following dental trauma are pain management and structural restoration, there is a growing understanding of how trauma can initiate or worsen periodontal disease. Injuries to the periodontal ligament and surrounding alveolar bone can impair the tooth's support system, leading to mobility, bone loss, and periodontal pocket formation over time A study by Andreasen et al. suggests that traumatic dental injuries can lead to increased susceptibility to periodontal disease due to alterations in the oral environment and potential disruption of normal oral hygiene practices [28]. Injuries can create areas where plaque accumulation is more likely, contributing to gingival inflammation and, if left untreated, progressing to periodontitis. 4-year retrospective study showed that following dental trauma, 62% of injured teeth had periodontal damage, and from this total, crown-root fractures with invasion of biological width were found in 42% of the cases, followed by bone injury (30%). Regarding the periodontal treatment performed, periodontal surgery to re-establish the biological width prevailed between procedures in 39% of the cases. When the biological width is invaded, an inflammatory reaction occurs on the periodontium, which causes alveolar bone resorption in order to generate more space for new connective tissue. Consequently, a deepening gingival groove is opened which can lead to chronic inflammation. The average of biologic width is established, as follows gingival sulcus: 0.69 mm; junctional epithelium: 0.97 mm; and connective tissue attachment: 1.07 mm. So, there is 2–3 mm of sound tooth structure coronal to the alveolar bone crest to the junctional epithelium and connective tissue attachment that can properly join the tooth. In these situations, the re-establishment of the biologic width with an increased clinical crown may be performed through surgical crown lengthening procedures and surgical or orthodontic extrusion, each one when properly indicated. The interplay between dental trauma and periodontal disease is complex. Trauma to the teeth and supporting structures can lead to direct damage to the periodontium, creating an environment conducive to bacterial colonization and inflammation. Conversely, the presence of periodontal disease can make teeth more susceptible to trauma due to the weakening of the supportive tissues.

Patients with periodontal disease have weakened support structures, making their teeth more vulnerable to trauma [29]. Additionally, periodontal inflammation can impair the healing process after a traumatic injury, further complicating recovery and leading to a cycle of worsening periodontal health and increased susceptibility to future trauma.

Occlusal trauma refers to damage caused by excessive or abnormal forces applied to the teeth during mastication or other parafunctional habits, such as bruxism. Unlike dental trauma caused by external forces, occlusal trauma results from internal dysfunctions, such as malocclusion or an improperly aligned bite. Occlusal trauma was defined as a co-destructive factor in the development of periodontal disease. Occlusal trauma can contribute to periodontal breakdown by increasing mechanical stress on the periodontium, leading to increased inflammation and accelerated tissue loss in the presence of bacterial plaque [28]. Research by Lammie et al. found that patients with significant occlusal trauma showed increased markers of periodontal inflammation, including elevated levels of gingival crevicular fluid and periodontal pocket depth [30]. This suggests that occlusal trauma can exacerbate periodontal conditions by increasing mechanical strain on periodontal tissues, thereby worsening gingivitis and periodontitis.

Psychological trauma resulting from dental and occlusal injuries can manifest as stress, anxiety, and depression. The psychological impact can influence oral health behaviors and biological responses that exacerbate periodontal conditions. Individuals experiencing psychological trauma may exhibit poorer oral hygiene practices due to decreased motivation or increased neglect of oral care routines. A study by Kiecolt-Glaser et al. found that stress and depression are associated with impaired immune responses and reduced adherence to oral hygiene practices, which can lead to increased risk of gingivitis and periodontitis [31]. Psychological stress affects the body's inflammatory response, which can exacerbate periodontal disease. Research by Chapple and Matthews indicated that stress can increase the production of pro-inflammatory cytokines, contributing to periodontal tissue breakdown and progression of periodontitis [32]. Genco et al. provided strong evidence linking psychological factors to periodontal disease, emphasizing that patients under stress are more prone to periodontal attachment loss. It was found that in the patients with periodontal disease, the level of anxiety was increased compared with periodontally healthy individuals [33]. Stress-related immune suppression, increased cortisol levels and poor oral hygiene habits are contributing factors in the development and progression of periodontitis.

Dental anxiety is a significant barrier to the effective management of both dental trauma and periodontal disease. Patients with dental anxiety are often reluctant to seek treatment, leading to delayed diagnosis and worsening of their conditions. The anxiety associated with dental visits is particularly pronounced in individuals who have experienced traumatic dental injuries or painful periodontal procedures in the past.

Studies have shown that dental anxiety is strongly associated with poor periodontal health outcomes. Anxious patients are less likely to adhere to regular dental visits and oral hygiene practices, leading to the progression of periodontal disease. Moreover, the fear of invasive procedures, such as scaling and root planning, can cause patients to avoid seeking treatment until the disease has advanced significantly.

7. Treatment strategies

Periodontal disease associated with dental trauma is a complex condition that requires a multidisciplinary approach, addressing both the periodontal and traumatic aspects.

In the case of TDI, immediate care is crucial. This includes repositioning displaced tooth/teeth, splinting, and maintaining oral hygiene to prevent secondary infection. Andreasen et al. [28] showed that early management of traumatic dental injury (TDI) significantly improved the healing of periodontal tissue and prevented further bone loss. Monitoring the periodontal status of injured teeth is a very important aspect of the management of the patient. If TDI results in the formation of deep pockets, nonsurgical therapy (scaling and root planning) will be required to reduce bacterial load.

Surgical treatment may be required to restore the affected structures. Surgery may include regenerative procedures, such as bone grafting or tissue grafting procedures, or crown lengthening and osseous surgeries to access healthy tooth structure and re-create biological width.

In case of the occlusal trauma, occlusal adjustment can help to redistribute forces and relieve strain on periodontal tissues. It can involve selective grinding of tooth surfaces or restoration of worn or broken teeth. Teeth with mobility due to occlusal trauma can be stabilized using splints, which helps to limit further mobility and trauma to the periodontal ligament. Orthodontic treatment can help to correct the misalignment of teeth that contributes to occlusal trauma. Harrel et al. [34] demonstrated that controlling occlusal trauma in conjunction with periodontal therapy can significantly reduce probing depth and improve attachment levels.

Stress reduction techniques, including counseling, meditation, and cognitive behavioral therapy can help mitigate the impact of psychological stress on oral health.

Since bruxism is often linked to psychological trauma, it can be managed with night guards to protect teeth and periodontium from excessive force. Educating patients on the importance of maintaining good oral hygiene despite psychological challenges is critical in preventing the progression of periodontal disease. In some cases, medications, like anxiolytics or antidepressants may be necessary to manage the psychological component contributing to periodontal disease. Effective management of dental anxiety requires a multifaceted approach, including behavioral interventions, sedation techniques, and building a trusting relationship between the patient and the dental care provider.

In modern days, access to innovative technologies helps to diagnose and treat periodontitis associated with dental trauma more efficiently and faster. For example, a three-dimensional image (Cone Beam CT) can help identify root fractures and the extent of destruction without the need for exploratory surgery. Laser technology has emerged as a valuable tool in the treatment of periodontal disease, especially for patients who have experienced dental trauma or suffer from anxiety. Its minimally invasive nature, precision, and ability to promote faster healing make it particularly advantageous for these patients [35, 36]. Key benefits of laser therapy include reduced bleeding and swelling, decontamination of periodontal pockets, promotion of tissue regeneration, sterilization of the treated areas, and fewer postoperative complications [37, 38]. By offering a more comfortable and efficient treatment experience, laser therapy not only improves clinical outcomes but also increases patient acceptance and adherence to necessary periodontal care [39]. Periodontitis in younger populations often requires long-term follow-up to prevent recurrence. Regular periodontal maintenance appointments, including professional cleanings and monitoring, are crucial to ensuring long-term stability.

7.1 Clinical recommendations

1. *Comprehensive assessment*: Dentists should assess both the physical and psychological impacts of trauma on oral health.

2. *Integrated care*: Collaboration with mental health professionals may be necessary to manage psychological trauma and its effects on oral health.

3. *Preventive measures*: Emphasize the importance of maintaining good oral hygiene and managing stress to prevent the progression of gingivitis and periodontitis.

8. Conclusion

The interrelationship between dental trauma, occlusal trauma, periodontal disease, and dental anxiety highlights the importance of a comprehensive and multidisciplinary approach to dental care. Dentists must be vigilant in identifying signs of trauma and periodontal disease, understanding how they can exacerbate each other, and addressing the psychological barriers that may prevent patients from seeking timely care, utilizing all the tools that modern dentistry can offer today.

Future research should focus on the long-term outcomes of patients who experience both dental trauma and periodontal disease, as well as developing new strategies to mitigate dental anxiety in this population. Understanding the complex interactions between these factors is essential for improving patient outcomes and maintaining optimal oral health.

Author details

Elena Furman
Department of Periodontology, Case Western Reserve University, School of Dental Medicine, Cleveland, Ohio, United States

*Address all correspondence to: exf19@case.edu

References

[1] Slots J. Periodontitis: Facts, fallacies and the future. Periodontology. 2017;**2000**(75):7-23

[2] Marcenes W et al. Global burden of periodontal disease in 2010 and its association with other diseases. Journal of Dental Research. 2013;**92**(11):865-871. DOI: 10.1177/0022034513502129

[3] Eke PI, Thornton-Evans GO, Wei L, et al. Periodontitis in US adults: National Health and nutrition examination survey 2009-2014. Journal of the American Dental Association (1939). 2018;**149**:576-588

[4] Eke PI et al. Prevalence of periodontitis in adults in the United States: 2009 and 2010. Journal of Dental Research. 2015;**94**(10):1435-1442. DOI: 10.1177/0022034515614276

[5] American Academy of Periodontology (AAP). Classification of periodontal and peri-implant diseases and conditions. Periodontology 2000. 2018;**76**(1):1-27. DOI: 10.1111/prd.12285

[6] Socransky SS, Haffajee AD, Cugini MA, et al. Microbial complexes in subgingival plaque. Journal of Clinical Periodontology. 1998;**25**:134-144

[7] Taubman MA, Valverde P, Han X, et al. Immune response: The key to bone resorption in periodontal disease. Journal of Periodontology. 2005;**76**(Suppl. 11):2033-2041

[8] Georgieva I. Trauma from occlusion—Types, clinical signs and clinical significance. A review. Scripta Scientifica Medicinae Dentalis. 2021;**7**(1):7-11

[9] Glickman I, Roeber F, Brion M, Pameijer JH. Photoelastic analysis of internal stresses in the periodontium created by occlusal forces. Journal of Periodontology. 1970;**41**(1):30-35. DOI: 10.1902/jop.1970.41.1.30

[10] Glickman I, Smulow J. Alterations in the pathway of gingival inflammation into the underlying tissues induced by excessive occlusal forces. Journal of Periodontology. 1962;**33**:7-13

[11] Jin LJ, Cao CF. Clinical diagnosis of trauma from occlusion and its relation with severity of periodontitis. Journal of Clinical Periodontology. 1992;**19**(2):92-97

[12] Fan J, Caton JG. Occlusal trauma and excessive occlusal forces: Narrative review, case definitions, and diagnostic considerations. Journal of Periodontology. 2018;**89**(Suppl. 1):S214-S222

[13] Polson AM, Meitner SW, Zander HA. Trauma and progression of marginal periodontitis in squirrel monkeys. III adaption of interproximal alveolar bone to repetitive injury. Journal of Periodontal Research. 1976;**11**(5):279-289

[14] Ramfjord SP, Kohler CA. Periodontal reaction to functional occlusal stress. Journal of Periodontology. 1959;**14**(30):95-112

[15] Kantor M, Polson AN, Zander HA. Alveolar bone regeneration after removal of inflammatory and traumatic factors. Journal of Periodontology. 1976;**47**(12):687-695

[16] Lam R. Epidemiology and outcomes of traumatic dental injuries: A review of the literature. Australian Dental Journal. 2016;**61**(Suppl. 1):4-20

[17] Kaste LM, Gift HC, Bhat M, Swango PA. Prevalence of incisor trauma in persons 6-50 years of age: United

States, 1988-1991. Journal of Dental Research. 1996;**75**:696-705

[18] Bastone E, Freer T, McNamara J. Epidemiology of dental trauma: A review of literature. Australian Dental Journal. 2000;**45**:2-9

[19] Andersson L. Epidemiology of traumatic dental injuries. Journal of Endodontia. 2013;**39**:2-5

[20] Glendor U. Epidemiology of traumatic dental injuries – A 12 year review of the literature. Dental Traumatology. 2008;**24**:603-611

[21] Kinjaric T, Leko J, Gorseta K. Dental anxiety in children in relation to dental health. Collegium Antropologicum. 2019;**43**:265-270

[22] Eklund M et al. The impact of dental trauma on psychological and social well-being. Community Dentistry and Oral Epidemiology. 2016;**44**(6):571-578

[23] Grembowski D et al. Dental trauma and PTSD: The psychological impact of oral injuries. Journal of Dental Research. 2019;**98**(6):683-690

[24] Mäki H et al. The relationship between dental trauma and depression in adults. Journal of Affective Disorders. 2018;**239**:30-37

[25] Kiecolt-Glaser JK et al. Psychological stress and the immune system: Role of periodontal disease. Psychosomatic Medicine. 2013;**75**(3):264-271

[26] Garcia RI et al. The impact of depression on periodontal health: A review. Journal of Periodontology. 2018;**89**(8):1005-1012

[27] Kvesic AJ et al. Possible risk factors for dental fear and anxiety in children who suffered traumatic dental injury. Dentistry Journal. 2023;**11**:190

[28] Andreasen JO, Andreasen FM, Andersson L. Traumatic Dental Injuries: A Manual. Willey Blackwell; 2007

[29] Lindhe J, Lang NP. Clinical Periodontology and Implant Dentistry. Blackwell Publishing; 2008

[30] Lammie G, Hughes FJ. Occlusal trauma and periodontal disease. Journal of Periodontology. 2014;**85**(1):1-11

[31] Kiecolt-Glaser JK, Glaser R. Psychological stress, immunity, and periodontal disease. Journal of Periodontology. 2013;**84**(2):262-274

[32] Chapple IL, Matthews JB. The role of inflammation in periodontal disease. Journal of Clinical Periodontology. 2007;**34**(1):16-21

[33] Genco RJ, Ho AW, Grossi SG, Dunford RG, Tedesco LA. Relationship of stress, distress, and inadequate coping behaviors to periodontal disease. Journal of Periodontology. 1999;**70**:711-723

[34] Harrel SK, Nunn ME. The effect of occlusal discrepancies on periodontitis. II. Relationship of occlusal treatment to the progression of periodontal disease; 2001. DOI: 10.1902/jop.2001.72.4.495

[35] Sgolastra F, Severino M, Gatto R, Monaco A. Effectiveness of laser therapy in periodontal disease: A systematic review and meta-analysis. Journal of Periodontology. 2013;**84**(7):790-800

[36] Dederich DN, Bushick RD. Lasers in dentistry: Separating science from hype. Journal of the American Dental Association. 2004;**135**(2):204-212

[37] Schwarz F, Aoki A, Becker J, Sculean A. Laser application in non-surgical periodontal therapy: A systematic review. Journal of Clinical Periodontology. 2008;**35**(S8):29-44

[38] Romanos GE, Nentwig GH. Diode laser (980 nm) in oral and maxillofacial

surgical procedures: Clinical observations based on clinical applications. Journal of Clinical Laser Medicine and Surgery. 2012;**16**(5):245-249

[39] Chikamatsu K, Kaneko N, Hirai M, Noguchi K. Patient satisfaction with laser therapy for periodontal disease: A questionnaire survey. Journal of Oral Laser Applications. 2008;**8**(4):243-248

Chapter 5

"Socket Oriented" Tooth Repositioning in Traumatic Dental Injuries

Tak On Ryan Tse

Abstract

Traumatic dental injuries, such as crown fractures, luxations, and avulsions, are common occurrences that can have significant consequences, including compromised esthetics, impaired function, and even tooth loss. Prompt and appropriate treatment is crucial for achieving favorable long-term outcomes, as recommended by the International Association of Dental Traumatology (IADT) guidelines. To address the challenge of accurately repositioning displaced teeth, the "socket oriented" tooth repositioning technique has been proposed. This method utilizes the alveolar socket as a guide, rather than solely relying on the patient's recollection, to enhance the precision of the repositioning process and improve clinical outcomes.

Keywords: dental trauma, luxations, avulsion, traumatic dental injuries, tooth repositioning, socket-oriented technique, splinting, International Association of Dental Traumatology (IADT)

1. Introduction

Traumatic dental injuries to permanent teeth are a common occurrence, with crown fractures, luxations, and avulsions being among the most frequently encountered types of traumas [1–3]. These types of injuries can have significant consequences, including compromised esthetics, impaired function, and even tooth loss if not properly managed.

Prompt and appropriate treatment of traumatic dental injuries is crucial for achieving favorable long-term outcomes. Treatment guidelines are well documented by the International Association of Dental Traumatology (IADT). The first set of guidelines was published in 2001 [4–8] and updated in 2007 [9–11], 2012 [12–15], and 2020 [16–18]. In the luxations and avulsion cases, tooth repositioning and splinting are recommended.

A key aspect of this treatment involves the precise repositioning of displaced teeth back into their original location within the alveolar socket [13, 14]. Accurate repositioning not only restores the tooth's proper alignment but also facilitates the healing process and helps maintain the overall integrity of the dentition.

 IntechOpen

However, accurately repositioning a displaced tooth can be challenging, particularly in cases where the patient is unable to clearly recall or convey the tooth's original position prior to the trauma. This can lead to malpositioning of the tooth, which can have detrimental effects on both esthetics and function [19, 20].

2. The "socket oriented" tooth repositioning technique

To address this common clinical challenge, the "socket oriented" tooth repositioning technique has been proposed as a reliable approach for restoring traumatized teeth to their proper position. By using the alveolar socket as a guide, rather than solely relying on the patient's recollection, this method aims to enhance the precision of the repositioning process and, ultimately, improve clinical outcomes.

The "socket oriented" repositioning technique for the management of traumatic dental injuries relies on the premise that the alveolar socket can serve as a reliable guide for accurately restoring the displaced tooth to its original position. This approach is particularly advantageous in cases where the patient's recollection of the pre-trauma tooth position is unclear or uncertain, a common scenario in the aftermath of a traumatic event.

The rationale behind this technique is based on the understanding that the alveolar socket is a three-dimensional structure that precisely matches the morphology of the tooth it houses. By carefully examining the socket, the clinician can assess the original orientation and inclination of the displaced tooth, providing valuable information to guide the repositioning process.

The step-by-step procedure for the "socket oriented" repositioning technique is as follows:

1. Careful examination of the tooth socket: The first critical step is to thoroughly examine the empty tooth socket to assess its original orientation and angulation. This can be done by visually inspecting the socket walls and noting any distinctive features or landmarks that may help determine the tooth's pre-trauma position.

2. Gentle repositioning of the displaced tooth: Once the original socket orientation has been determined, the displaced tooth can be gently repositioned back into the socket. The clinician should aim to align the tooth with the walls of the socket, ensuring that it is seated in its proper position and relationship with the surrounding dentition.

3. Patient positioning: To facilitate the repositioning process and ensure optimal visibility, the patient should be positioned at a 45-degree angle. This position can help prevent the lower mandible from dropping back and also allow the patient to move the lower jaw and test the functional envelope (**Figures 1** and **2**). The clinician should place a finger on the tooth and ask the patient to move the lower jaw inside out while in function. There should not be crepitus when the tooth is in function (**Figure 3**).

4. Splint the tooth with the adjacent tooth: The use of passive and flexible splints for the stabilization of traumatized teeth is recommended. Commonly used materials include 0.4 mm diameter stainless steel wire or nylon fishing line, which are

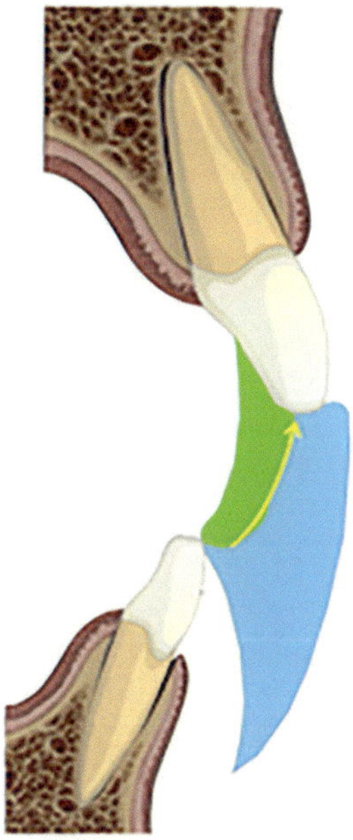

Figure 1.
When the patient is lying in the supine (back) position, the lower jaw (mandible) drops back and posteriorly. The green line indicates the range of motion and movement of the mandible in this supine position. The blue shaded area represents the functional envelope—The maximum opening and range of motion the jaw can achieve in this reclined posture.

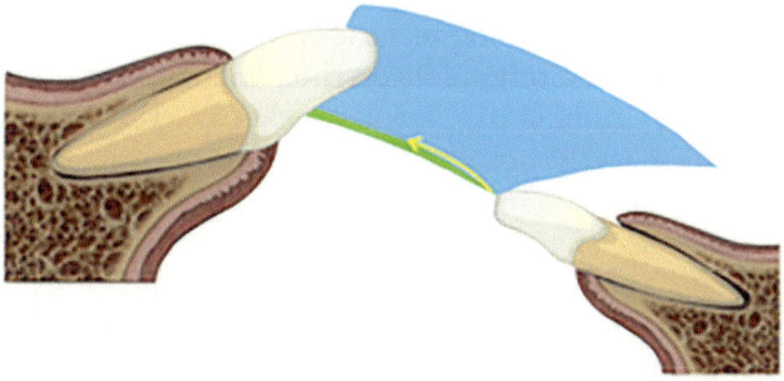

Figure 2.
When the patient is seated in an upright position, the lower jaw position and range of motion changes significantly. The green line now shows a different, more forward pathway of mandibular movement compared to the supine position. The blue functional envelope is also altered, likely increasing in size and shifting forward when the patient is upright.

bonded to the teeth using composite resin. These splints allow for some degree of mobility, which is crucial for the healing process, while still providing the necessary support and stabilization [21–24].

5. Occlusion checking: After the tooth has been splinted, the clinician should use 200-micron articulating paper to check the occlusal contacts while the patient is functioning. Make sure that there is no ink streak in the functional path. This step is crucial to ensure that the repositioned tooth is in proper functional alignment with the opposing dentition, minimizing the risk of subsequent trauma or complications.

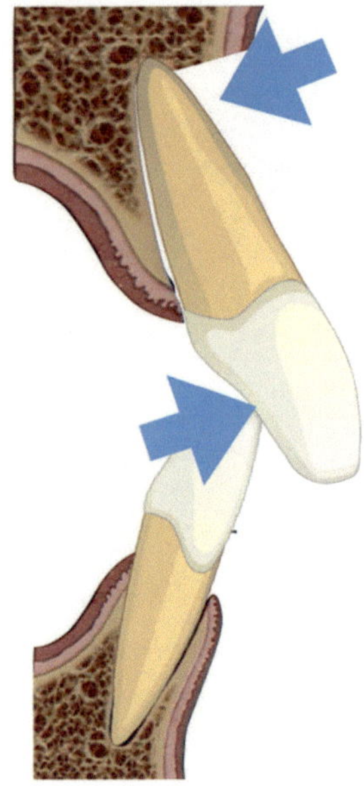

Figure 3.
The diagram illustrates the "socket-oriented" repositioning technique. The clinician uses their fingers to palpate the root apex and reposition it back into the proper socket. Simultaneously, the crown is positioned based on the reference of the lower teeth. The patient is seated in a 45-degree reclined position, ensuring that the mandible is moved within the functional envelope during the repositioning.

2.1 Advantages of the "socket oriented" technique

The "socket oriented" repositioning technique offers several key advantages over traditional approaches that rely solely on the patient's recollection of the pre-trauma tooth position. By utilizing the alveolar socket as a reliable anatomical guide, this method helps to improve the accuracy of the repositioning process, leading to enhanced esthetic and functional outcomes for the patient.

Furthermore, the precise alignment of the tooth within the socket can contribute to improved healing and a reduced risk of long-term complications, such as ankylosis or root resorption. This is particularly important in the management of traumatic dental injuries, where the preservation of the natural dentition is a primary treatment goal.

In this chapter, we will explore the rationale, methodology, and clinical applications of the "socket oriented" tooth repositioning technique in the management of traumatic dental injuries. Through the presentation of illustrative case examples, we will demonstrate the effectiveness of this approach in restoring both the esthetic and functional integrity of the dentition following various types of traumatic injuries.

The case presented highlights the complexities involved in the management of traumatic dental injuries, particularly in situations where multiple teeth are affected, and the patient's treatment preferences need to be carefully considered.

2.2 Treatment case 1

The 40-year-old female patient sustained significant trauma, as she lost consciousness and fell onto the table, resulting in fractures of 11, 12, severe intrusion, and lateral subluxation of 21 and 22.

2.2.1 Clinical exam

Tooth 11 was RCT treated and crown-root fractures extend below the gingival margin in the palatal side (**Figure 4**).

Tooth 21 was severely injured with lateral and intrusive luxation.

Tooth 22 had lateral luxation.

The comprehensive assessment of the patient's condition, including the use of advanced imaging techniques such as cone beam computed tomography (CBCT), was crucial in formulating an appropriate treatment plan [25, 26]. It gives detail information about the 3D position of the tooth. The intraoral 2D radiographs cannot reveal the severity of the injury. It cannot show the displacement of the root and also the alveolar fracture.

2.2.2 Treatment plan

The CBCT findings (**Figures 5–7**) provided crucial insights into the extent and severity of the injuries sustained by the patient. The intrusion and labial placement of tooth 21, coupled with the labial plate fracture, presented a significant challenge. Similarly, the lateral luxation of tooth 22 and the widening of the lamina dura indicated the need for a thorough assessment and a carefully considered treatment plan.

In formulating the treatment options, the clinician's discussions with the patient were of paramount importance. By thoroughly explaining the potential complications and the prognosis associated with each treatment approach, the clinician ensured that the patient was well-informed and could make a decision that aligned with their preferences and expectations [27–29].

For tooth 11, the treatment options included crown lengthening, fiber post, and a full ceramic crown, or extraction and replacement with an implant. The clinician's evaluation of the extent of the crown-root fracture below the gingival margin likely guided the decision to consider these alternatives, as the restoration of the tooth needed to address the compromised tooth structure and achieve an optimal esthetic outcome.

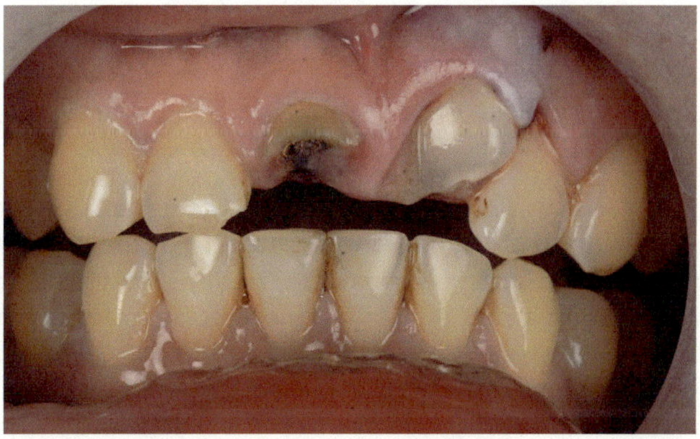

Figure 4.
The pre-operative photo: Tooth 11 was fractured and extended below the gingival margin on the palatal side. Tooth 21 was severely injured, with both lateral and intrusive luxation. Tooth 22 had lateral luxation.

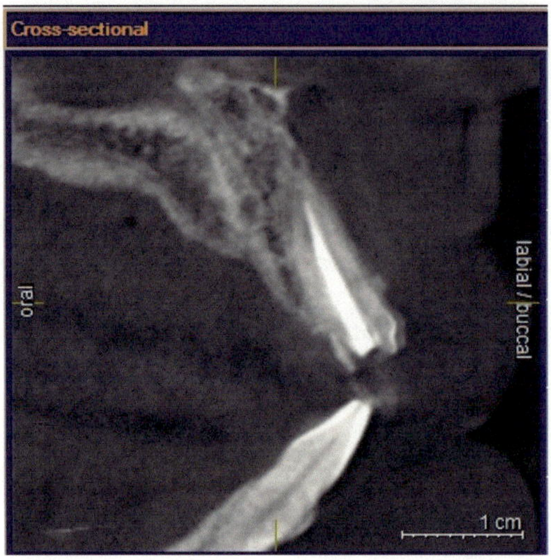

Figure 5.
CBCT of tooth 11 shows it was root canal treated, with a crown-root fracture extending below the gingival margin on the palatal (palatal) side.

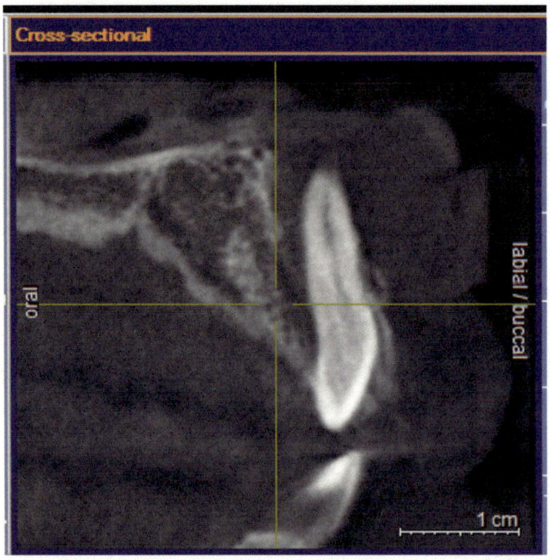

Figure 6.
CBCT of tooth 21 shows it was intruded and displaced labially, with a fracture of the labial bone plate. The tooth apex is also positioned labially.

The more complex scenario presented by tooth 21 required a nuanced approach. The clinician's recognition that the extraction of this tooth could lead to severe bone resorption and poor esthetic outcomes was a crucial consideration. Given the patient's interest in preserving their natural dentition, the decision to attempt tooth repositioning and splinting was a strategic one. This approach aimed to stabilize the tooth, facilitate healing, and potentially maintain the alveolar architecture, thereby preserving the foundation for future restorative options, should the need arise.

The clinician's thoughtful consideration of the patient's preferences, the potential complications, and the long-term prognosis demonstrated a comprehensive and patient-centric approach to the management of this traumatic dental injury. By thoroughly

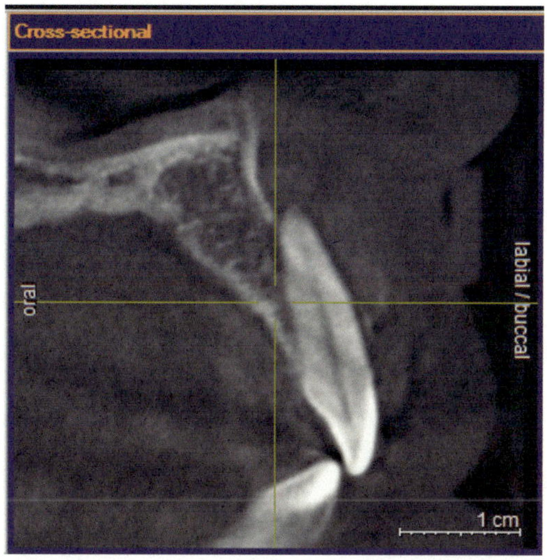

Figure 7.
CBCT of tooth 22 demonstrates lateral luxation. The lamina dura (bony socket outline) appears widened.

discussing the treatment options and their implications, the clinician empowered the patient to make an informed decision that aligned with their values and goals.

2.2.3 Emergency treatment

The initial emergency treatment focused on the immediate stabilization of the affected teeth and restoration of the patient's smile. Tooth 21, which had experienced severe intrusion and lateral subluxation, was carefully repositioned using extraction forceps and then splinted together with the adjacent teeth. The clinician was informed that the patient's front teeth were well-aligned prior to the accident, and the clinician then positioned teeth 21 and 22 according to the patient's preference, using digital tools. Teeth 21–23 were then splinted with a fiber splint and composite material. The splint was placed in the middle of the teeth, away from the gingiva (**Figure 8**).

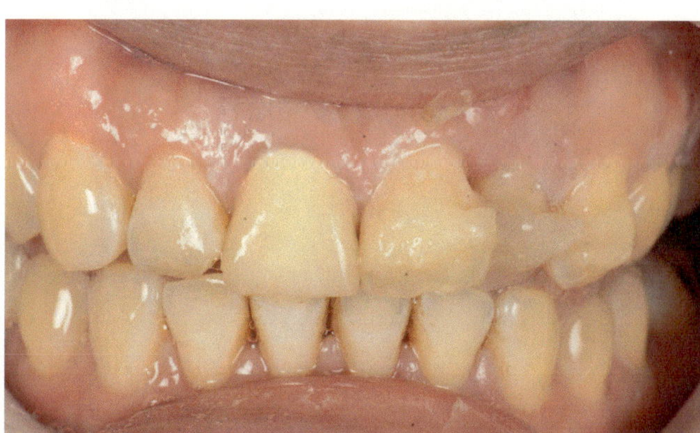

Figure 8.
Immediate post-splint photo. A temporary ceramic crown was placed on tooth 11. Teeth 21-23 were splinted together using a fiber-reinforced composite splint.

The patient was instructed to consume a soft diet for 2 weeks [30] and to avoid using the traumatized teeth while eating. Meticulous oral hygiene and the use of chlorhexidine mouth rinse was also recommended.

For tooth 11, a fiber post was placed, and an immediate temporary crown was milled using CEREC technology.

The splint was removed 8 weeks later. New CBCT was taken and the root apex of 21, 22 were labially placed (**Figures 9** and **10**). The teeth 21 and 22 were not positioned correctly due to the misleading information by the patient. Orthodontic treatment was advised to reposition the roots of 21 and 22 and also the extrusion of 11 for the ferrule effect of the restoration.

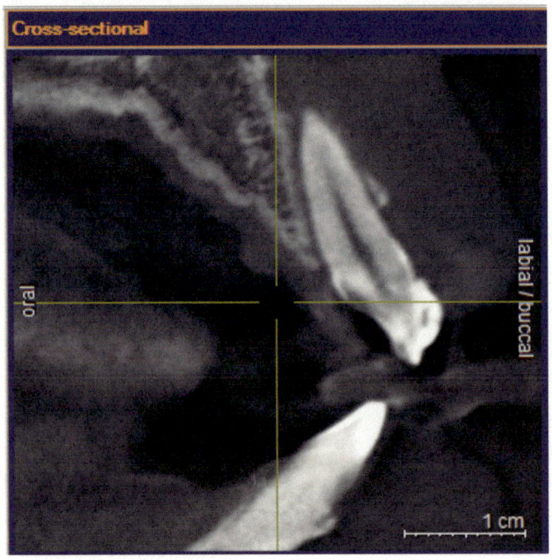

Figure 9.
Post-operative CBCT of tooth 21 shows the root apex was labially positioned, outside of the labial bone plate.

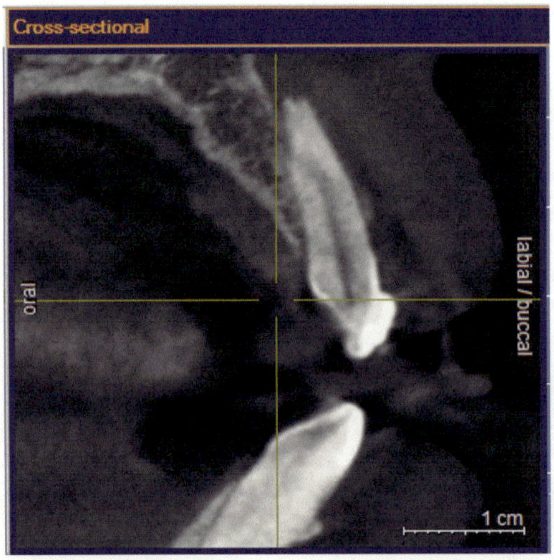

Figure 10.
CBCT of tooth 22 also shows the root apex was labially positioned.

But it was unfortunately declined by the patient: The crown lengthening procedure and the placement of a layered lithium disilicate crown on tooth 11 to achieve an optimal esthetic and functional outcome.

2.2.4 Review

The splint was removed 8 weeks after the initial treatment. A new CBCT was taken, which revealed that the root apices of teeth 21 and 22 were labially placed. The teeth were not positioned correctly, likely due to the misleading information provided by the patient. Orthodontic treatment was advised to reposition the roots of teeth 21 and 22, as well as to extrude tooth 11 for the ferrule effect of the restoration.

Unfortunately, the patient declined the orthodontic treatment. As a result, the clinician proceeded with a crown lengthening procedure and the placement of a layered lithium disilicate crown on tooth 11, in order to achieve an optimal esthetic and functional outcome (**Figure 11**). Teeth 21 and 22 had the root canal treatment due to the pulp necrosis after the trauma.

During the review, the patient continued to complain about discomfort in teeth 21 and 22, as well as headaches. Upon intraoral examination, the teeth were found to be slightly palatally inclined, which resulted in premature contact when the patient was eating. Crepitus was also detected on teeth 21 and 22.

The patient was asked to bite on 200-μm-thick articulating paper (Bausch) and bring the posterior teeth together into maximum intercuspation. This revealed blue streaks on the palatal surfaces of teeth 21 and 22, indicating interference in the functional pathways [31].

To address this issue, the clinician positioned the patient in an upright seated position and adjusted the lingual contours of the maxillary incisors until the marking ink no longer showed surface streaks during biting. After this adjustment, the crepitus was resolved, and the patient reported feeling better.

2.3 Case 2

The 65-year-old patient had sustained severe trauma to her upper jaw, with tooth 21 suffering from lateral and intrusive luxation (**Figure 12**). This type of injury

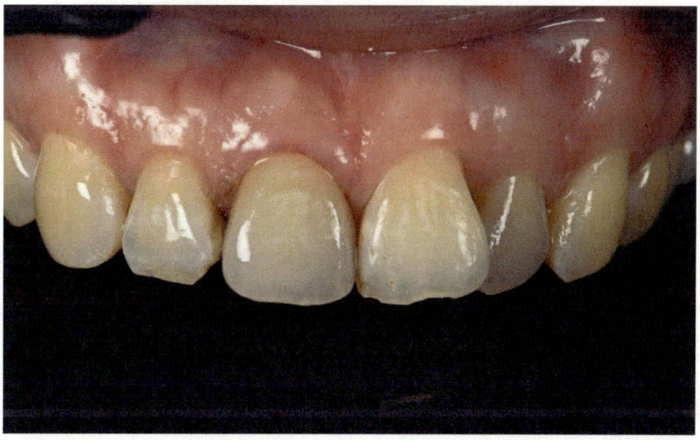

Figure 11.
Post-operative photo show the lithium disilicate crown 11 was cemented after the splint removal. The soft tissue healing appears excellent.

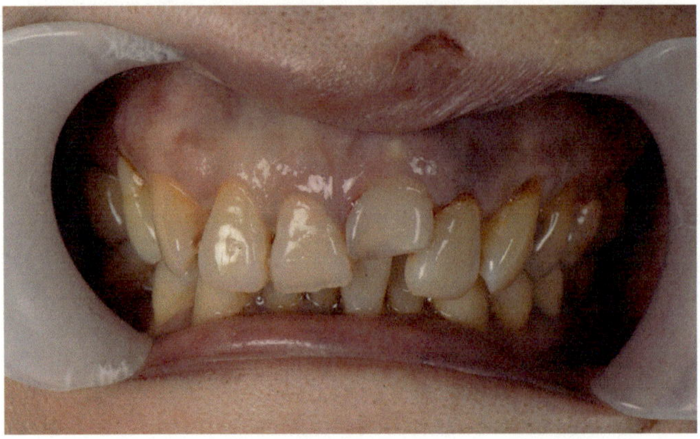

Figure 12.
Pre-operative photo—Tooth 21 had severe lateral and intrusive luxation injuries.

is challenging, as the tooth is not only displaced laterally but also intruded into the alveolar socket, with the root apex displaced labially and the labial bone plate fractured.

2.3.1 Treatment plan

The CBCT imaging was crucial in assessing the full extent of the injury. The CBCT scans clearly showed the severe intrusion of tooth 21, with the root apex displaced labially and the labial bone plate fractured. Additionally, tooth 22 was found to be palatally displaced with lateral luxation, and its labial bone plate was also fractured (**Figures 13** and **14**).

Given the severity of the injuries, the treatment planning was done in close consultation with the patient, thoroughly discussing the possible complications and

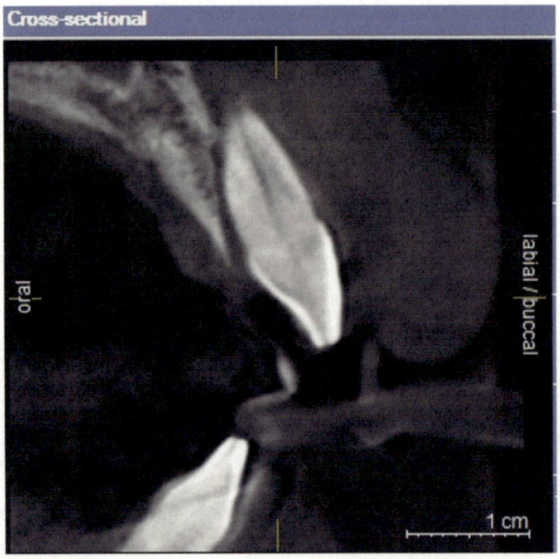

Figure 13.
Pre-operative CBCT of tooth 21 shows severe intrusion with the root apex displaced labially and the labial bone plate fractured.

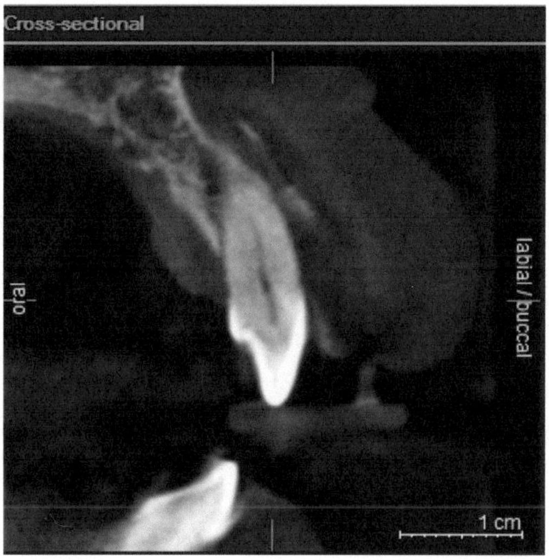

Figure 14.
Pre-operative CBCT of tooth 22 shows palatal displacement with lateral luxation, as well as a fracture of the labial bone plate.

prognosis [28–30]. The tooth was planned to reposition and splint and reviewed after 8 weeks. The possibility of root canal therapy was addressed. This collaborative approach is essential, as it ensures the patient is fully informed and engaged in the decision-making process.

2.3.2 Emergency treatment

The emergency treatment involved using a "socket-oriented" repositioning technique. Tooth 21 was gently extruded using extraction forceps. The clinician then used their index finger to palpate the apex of tooth 21 while the patient was in occlusion, allowing them to digitally reposition the root with reference to the labial plate of the adjacent teeth. They then pressed the root against the socket wall and used another finger to position the crown of tooth 21 in alignment with the adjacent teeth. This meticulous repositioning was crucial to ensure the tooth was properly aligned and stable within the socket.

In addition to the positioning of tooth 21 in the socket, the clinician needed to ensure that the tooth was positioned properly outside the chewing envelope. The patient was seated at a 45-degree angle and asked to protrude the mandible and then slide it back. The clinician felt for crepitus and made sure the tooth was positioned correctly without any crepitus during function. The tooth was then splinted with a fiber splint and composite. The splinting not only holds the tooth in place during the initial healing process but also allows for functional evaluation. After the splinting, the clinician used 200-micron articulating paper to check the occlusion and ensure there were no ink streaks on the palatal side [32].

2.3.3 Review

After 8 weeks, the splint was removed (**Figure 15**), and a new CBCT scan was obtained. The CBCT findings were encouraging, as they revealed that the root of

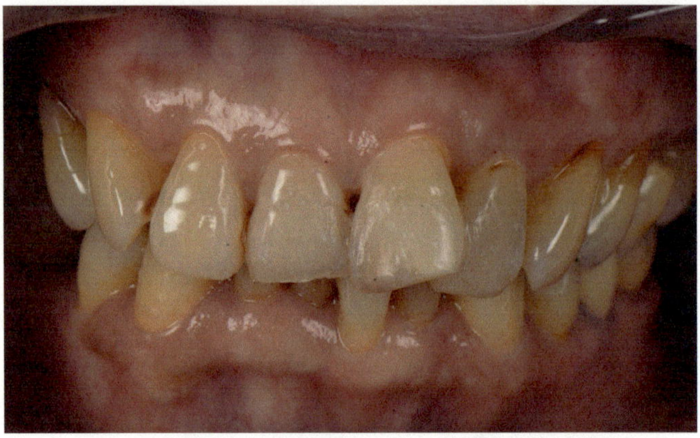

Figure 15.
Post-operative photo after splint removal. The teeth were aligned with the "socket oriented" tooth positioning technique and the crown were not well aligned, but were repositioned back to their original positions.

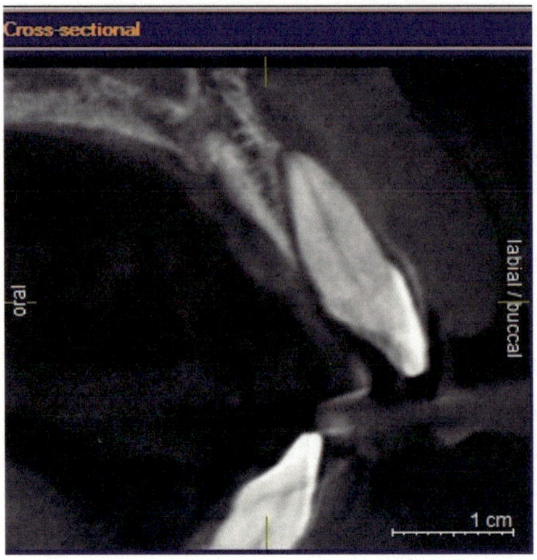

Figure 16.
CBCT 8 weeks post-operatively—Tooth 21 is well-aligned with the alveolar.

tooth 21 had healed well and was in a favorable position, suggesting a positive prognosis for the patient's long-term oral health (**Figure 16**).

3. Discussion

In the first clinical case, teeth 21 and 22 were positioned too retroclined, resulting in premature contact on the upper palatal surface and improper positioning of the teeth. The patient was advised to undergo orthodontic treatment but refused. Instead, the clinician opted for occlusal adjustment of the palatal surfaces of teeth 11, 21, and 22 to settle the occlusion. From the postoperative CBCT imaging, it was evident that the root apices were positioned labially, outside the labial bone plate. This highlights the importance of positioning the tooth from the root, rather than solely focusing on the crown position. The crown-focused approach was misleading, as the patient

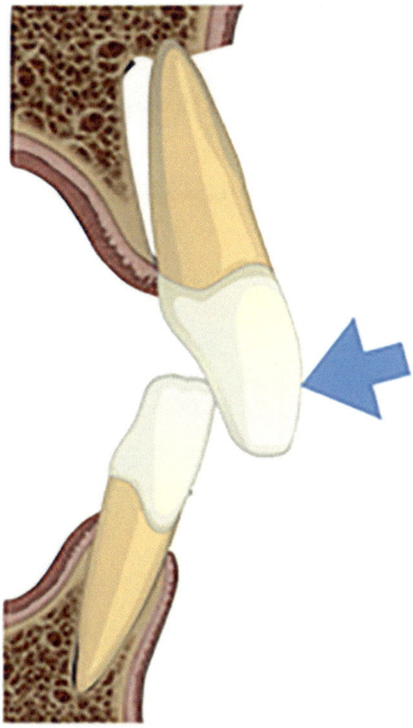

Figure 17.
This image illustrates the "crown-focus approach". The tooth was positioned in a retroclined orientation. The root apex was positioned outside of the tooth socket. This approach can affect the healing process and long-term prognosis of the tooth.

claimed that the tooth was well-aligned before, which resulted in the retroclined position (**Figure 17**). Failure to correctly reposition the tooth led to premature contact when the patient was in function (**Figure 18**).

In the worst-case scenario where the root apices of the retroclined teeth (21 and 22) were positioned outside the labial bone plate, there are several significant concerns:

1. Compromised bone support: With the root apices situated outside the bony housing, the long-term stability and health of these teeth are greatly jeopardized. The lack of adequate bone support around the root apices leaves them vulnerable to further displacement, resorption, and potential loss of the teeth.

2. Increased risk of gingival recession: The improper positioning of the root apices in relation to the bony housing can lead to thinning of the overlying gingiva and an increased risk of gingival recession. This can result in exposed root surfaces, compromised esthetics, and heightened sensitivity.

3. Impaired periodontal attachment: Without the proper bony support, the periodontal ligament and attachment fibers may be compromised, leading to a weakened connection between the tooth and the surrounding alveolar bone. This can increase the susceptibility to periodontal disease and further bone loss over time.

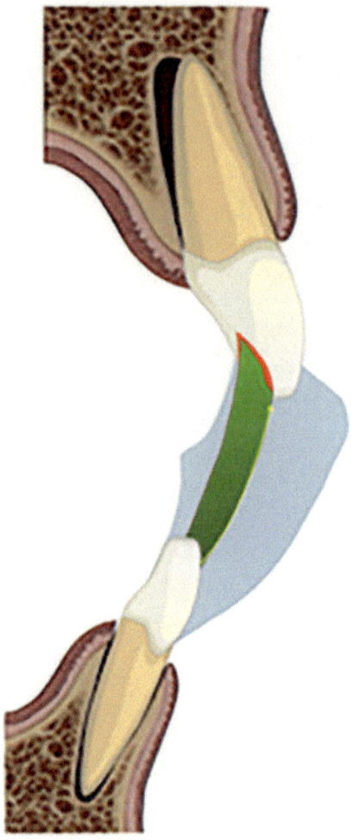

Figure 18.
This image also illustrates the "crown-focus approach". This resulted in premature contact when the patient was in function (occlusion). The red area indicates the heavy contact zone during function.

4. Biomechanical disadvantage: The retroclined position of the teeth and the lack of adequate bone support can create an unfavorable biomechanical environment. This can lead to increased stress on the teeth, the surrounding bone, and the overall periodontium during functional loading, further exacerbating the prognosis.

5. Difficulty in orthodontic correction: Attempting to orthodontically reposition these teeth may prove challenging, as the lack of bone support and the compromised periodontal attachment can limit the ability to move the teeth into a more favorable position.

In such a worst-case scenario, the long-term prognosis of these teeth becomes guarded, and the risk of complications, such as tooth loss or the need for more extensive restorative and/or surgical interventions, increases significantly. Immediate CBCT imaging is crucial in these cases to accurately assess the precise position of the root apices and develop an appropriate treatment plan to address the underlying issues and optimize the chances of a favorable outcome.

However, it is acknowledged that 3D imaging may not always be available in all clinical settings. In such situations, the clinician must rely on their clinical skills and expertise to enhance the diagnosis and treatment approach. Digital palpation is a valuable skill that can be employed in these cases. The clinician can use their index finger to palpate the apex of the traumatized tooth and the adjacent labial bone plate. This tactile examination allows the clinician to assess the displacement of the root apex and any potential fractures of the alveolar process. The technique names as socket oriented tooth positioning.

In the second clinical case, the clinician utilized a "socket-oriented" approach to reposition the tooth and then applied a splint. The postoperative CBCT findings revealed that the root was well-aligned and positioned, and the patient did not experience any discomfort in the occlusion. This technique of "socket-oriented" repositioning is particularly useful in ensuring the tooth is positioned in its natural, optimal position, which can greatly benefit the healing process and long-term prognosis of the tooth.

The use of 200-micron articulating paper to check the occlusion and ensure the teeth are positioned within the functional envelope is an important step in this treatment approach [32]. This meticulous evaluation helps to identify and address any premature contacts or interference, further enhancing the stability and long-term prognosis of the repositioned tooth.

In the current digital era, where patients, especially younger generations, frequently take selfie photographs, these can be a valuable clinical record for the clinician. The pre-trauma position of the tooth can be assessed using these visual references, which can guide the clinician in the repositioning and splinting procedures.

4. Conclusion

In conclusion, the use of 3D imaging, such as CBCT, is essential for the accurate diagnosis and treatment planning of dental trauma cases. However, when such advanced imaging is not readily available, the clinician must rely on their clinical skills and expertise, including digital palpation and utilization of patient-provided visual references, to guide the repositioning and stabilization of the traumatized teeth. The "socket-oriented" approach has demonstrated positive outcomes in managing complex dental injuries and restoring the patient's long-term oral health.

Author details

Tak On Ryan Tse
Restorative Dental Sciences, Faculty of Dentistry, University of Hong Kong, Hong Kong, China

*Address all correspondence to: tsetakon@hotmail.com

References

[1] International Association of Dental Traumatology. Dental trauma guidelines. Dental Traumatology. 2012;**28**(2):2-12

[2] Andreasen JO, Andreasen FM, Andersson L. Textbook and Color Atlas of Traumatic Injuries to the Teeth. 4th ed. Hoboken, New Jersey: Wiley-Blackwell; 2007

[3] Glendor U. Epidemiology of traumatic dental injuries—A 12 year review of the literature. Dental Traumatology. 2008;**24**(6):603-611

[4] Flores MT, Andreasen JO, Bakland LK, Feiglin B, Gutmann JL, Oikarinen K, et al. Guidelines for the evaluation and management of traumatic dental injuries (part l of the series). Dental Traumatology. 2001;**17**:1-4

[5] Flores MT, Andreasen JO, Bakland LK, Feiglin B, Gutmann JL, Oikarinen K, et al. Guidelines for the evaluation and management of traumatic dental injuries (part 2 of the series). Dental Traumatology. 2001;**17**:49-52

[6] Flores MT, Andreasen JO, Bakland LK, Feiglin B, Gutmann JL, Oikarinen K, et al. Guidelines for the evaluation and management of traumatic dental injuries (part 3 of the series). Dental Traumatology. 2001;**17**:97-102

[7] Flores MT, Andreasen JO, Bakland LK, Feiglin B, Gutmann JL, Oikarinen K, et al. Guidelines for the evaluation and management of traumatic dental injuries (part 4 of the series). Dental Traumatology. 2001;**17**:145-148

[8] Flores MT, Andreasen JO, Bakland LK, Feiglin B, Gutmann JL, Oikarinen K, et al. Guidelines for the evaluation and management of traumatic dental injuries (part 5 of the series). Dental Traumatology. 2001;**17**:193-198

[9] Flores MT, Andersson L, Andreasen JO, Bakland LK, Malmgren B, Barnett F, et al. Guidelines for the management of traumatic dental injuries. 1. Fractures and luxations of permanent teeth. Dental Traumatology. 2007;**23**:66-71

[10] Flores MT, Andersson L, Andreasen JO, Bakland LK, Malmgren B, Barnett F, et al. Guidelines for the management of traumatic dental injuries. 11. Avulsion of permanent teeth. Dental Traumatology. 2007;**23**:130-136

[11] Flores MT, Malmgren B, Andersson L, Andreasen JO, Bakland LK, Barnett F, et al. Guidelines for the management of traumatic dental injuries. 111. Primary teeth. Dental Traumatology. 2007;**23**:196-202

[12] Anderasen et al. International Association of Dental Traumatology guidelines for the management of traumatic dental injuries: 1. Fractures and luxations of permanent teeth. Dental Traumatology. 2012;**28**:2-12

[13] Andersson L, Andreasen JO, Day P, et al. International Association of Dental Traumatology guidelines for the management of traumatic dental injuries: 2. Avulsion of permanent teeth. Dental Traumatology. 2012;**28**:88-96. DOI: 10.1111/j.1600-9657.2012.01125.x

[14] Malmgren et al. International Association of Dental Traumatology guidelines for the management of traumatic dental injuries: 3. Injuries in the primary dentition. Dental Traumatology. 2012;**28**:174-182

[15] Levin L, Day PF, Hicks L, et al. International Association of Dental Traumatology guidelines for the management of traumatic dental injuries: General introduction. Dental Traumatology. 2020;**36**:309-313

[16] Bourguignon C, Cohenca N, Lauridsen E, et al. International Association of Dental Traumatology guidelines for the management of traumatic dental injuries: 1. Fractures and luxations. Dental Traumatology. 2020;**36**:314-330

[17] Andreasen JO, Andreasen FM. Textbook and Color Atlas of Traumatic Injuries to the Teeth. 3rd ed. Munksgaard, Copenhagen; 1994

[18] Flores MT, Andersson L, Andreasen JO, et al. Guidelines for the management of traumatic dental injuries. I. Fractures and luxations of permanent teeth. Dental Traumatology. 2007;**23**(2):66-71

[19] Fouad AF, Abbott PV, Tsilingaridis G, et al. International Association of Dental Traumatology guidelines for the management of traumatic dental injuries: 2. Avulsion of permanent teeth. Dental Traumatology. 2020;**36**:331-342

[20] Day P, Flores MT, O'Connell A, et al. International Association of Dental Traumatology guidelines for the management of traumatic dental injuries: 3. Injuries in the primary dentition. Dental Traumatology. 2020;**36**:343-359

[21] Kwan SC, Johnson JD, Cohenca N. The effect of splint material and thickness on tooth mobility after extraction and replantation using a human cadaveric model. Dental Traumatology. 2012;**28**:277-281

[22] Kahler B, Heithersay GS. An evidence-based appraisal of splinting luxated, avulsed and rootfractured teeth. Dental Traumatology. 2008;**24**:2-10

[23] Oikarinen K, Andreasen JO, Andreasen FM. Rigidity of various fixation methods used as dental splints. Endodontics & Dental Traumatology. 1992;**8**:113-119

[24] Andreasen JO, Andreasen FM, Mejare I, Cvek M. Healing of 400 intra-alveolar root fractures. 2. Effect of treatment factors such as treatment delay, repositioning, splinting type and period and antibiotics. Dental Traumatology. 2004;**20**:203-211

[25] Cohenca N, Silberman A. Contemporary imaging for the diagnosis and treatment of traumatic dental injuries: A review. Dental Traumatology. 2017;**33**:321-328

[26] Cohenca N, Simon JH, Mathur A, Malfaz JM. Clinical indications for digital imaging in dento-alveolar trauma. Part 2: Root resorption. Dental Traumatology. 2007;**23**:105-113

[27] Cohenca N, Simon JH, Roges R, Morag Y, Malfaz JM. Clinical indications for digital imaging in dento-alveolar trauma. Part 1: Traumatic injuries. Dental Traumatology. 2007;**23**:95-104

[28] Moule A, Cohenca N. Emergency assessment and treatment planning for traumatic dental injuries. Australian Dental Journal. 2016;**61**(Suppl. 1):21-38

[29] Andreasen FM, Andreasen JO, Tsukiboshi M, Cohenca N. Examaination and diagnosis of dental injuries. In: Andreasen JO, Andreasen FM, Andersson L, editors. Textbook and Color Atlas of Traumatic Injuries to the Teeth. 5th ed. Oxford: Wiley Blackwell; 2019. pp. 295-326

[30] Andreasen JO, Bakland L, Flores MT, Andreasen FM, Andersson L. Traumatic dental injuries. A manual. 3rd ed. Chichester, West Sussex: Wiley-Blackwell; 2011

[31] Andersson L, Lindskog S, Blomlof L, Hedstrom KG, Hammarstrom L. Effect of masticatory stimulation on dentoalveolar ankylosis after experimental tooth replantation. Endodontics & Dental Traumatology. 1985;**1**:13-16

[32] Bakeman EM, Kois JC. The myth of anterior guidance: 10 steps in designing proper clearance for functional pathways. Journal of Cosmetic Dentistry. 2012;**28**(3):56-62

Chapter 6

Effectiveness of Oral Splints in Temporomandibular Disorders

Ronald Roossevelt Ramos-Montiel,
Genesis Aileen Gordillo-Renteria, Lorenzo Puebla-Ramos,
Sergio Oscar-Palmas, Lorena Alexandra Gonzalez-Campoverde,
María Isabel Cabrera-Padrón,
Jessika Yesenia Rodriguez-Cumbicus
and Fernanda Gabriela Carmona-Barreto

Abstract

Temporomandibular joint (TMJ) is one of the most complex structures of the human body because it allows opening and closing movements and in turn slides forward, backward, and laterally during the physiological functions of the cranio-cervico-maxillo-facial region. However, the parafunctions and/or exaggerated functions could generate wear on the structures that conform to it and on which its balance is based, generating temporomandibular disorders (TMD). These are observed through a peculiar semiology in which predominate the limitations of the mandibular movements accompanied by pain. The prevalence of TMD is remarkably high, affecting between 15 and 40% of the world population. Some studies suggest that the incidence could be higher due to unreported cases. Treatment for TMD is multidisciplinary and focuses on jaw stabilization with redistribution of forces and prevention of bruxism, for which the most popular method described is oral splints, with divided criteria about their efficacy; therefore, the question arises to what extent oral splints improve quality of life and reduce symptoms in patients with TMD.

Keywords: efficiency, oral splints, splint therapy, temporomandibular disorder, temporomandibular joint

1. Introduction

Temporomandibular disorder (TMD) is characterized by clinical problems that mainly affect the temporomandibular joint, as well as the myofascial muscles and associated structures. It is mentioned that it has come to alter the neuromuscular system; however, these could cause pain of non-dental origin in the orofacial region, including the head, face, and structures of the maxillofacial cranio-cervical region [1–5].

IntechOpen

The temporomandibular joint (TMJ) is formed by the mandibular condyle and the glenoid surface of the temporal bone; these two bones are separated by the articular disc. In turn, the articular portion of the articular disc is composed of fibrous connective tissue, nerves, vessels, and synovial fluid, which is attached to the bony structures by collateral ligaments. This synovial fluid helps in the articular movement, the transport of nutrients, and the disposal of the articular surfaces during its operation [5–10].

Patients with TMD could have problems, especially in their quality of life, having a negative result in their eating and speech. It also causes muscle sensitivity to palpation, restriction of the mouth opening, myogenic pain, pain and noise in the TMJ, orofacial pain located on the regions of the masseter, and anterior temporal muscle, and in some cases, has presented pain in the ear and neck, musculoskeletal disorders of the cervical spine, dizziness, and burning tongue. For this reason, in 2020, between 5 and 12% of the global population could have experienced some type of sign or symptom of temporomandibular disorder, making it the second most common cause of facial pain [3, 11–14].

During mastication, the tolerance of the articular physiological limit could be exceeded due to several circumstances; therefore, an overexertion of the compensatory capacities of the masticatory and neuromuscular systems is produced, which would lead to a rupture of the balance and functionality, and there would also be a minimum risk factor caused by psychological factors and genetics. In other words, functional overload, trauma, joint disease, and increased friction between the moving parts play an important role as they may lead to a displacement of the articular disc and consequently the establishment and development of TMD [3, 6, 15, 16].

Until the beginning of the twentieth century, the treatment of TMD was mainly based on the use of oral splints, including non-invasive approaches such as physiotherapy, education, behavioral counseling, relaxation therapy, and minimally invasive systems (pharmacological intervention and arthroscopic surgery). First of all, it was important to perform an initial radiograph, in which the radiolucent joint space between the mandibular condyle and the articular bone would be observed. These oral splints are recognized to be a non-surgical method with more effectiveness because it would help in sleep apnea, successfully reduce discomfort and pain-related disability, and increase coping skills by improving cognitions and adaptive behaviors; however, oral splints could be used between 6 weeks and 3 months [1, 4, 15, 17–20].

For this reason, and for clinical updates on the use of oral splints, the present study sought to know if there are other treatments for temporomandibular joint injuries and the effectiveness of oral splints in the treatment of TMD.

2. TMJ disorders: diagnosis, symptoms, and contributing factors

Everyone may experience pain in the orofacial region, which may possibly be transitory and associated with some disease, but in some cases, such pain may be chronic, so a correct diagnosis and treatment will be needed based on the symptomatology and clinical picture of orofacial pain [21].

TMD is defined as the second most common origin of orofacial pain, involving the muscles of mastication, the temporomandibular joint, and associated structures; therefore, it is mainly characterized by affecting the temporomandibular joint area, the muscles of the face, mastication, and ear. In addition, there are other signs and symptoms, such as clicking in the joints, limited opening of the mouth, and palpation. These symptoms could cause future damage to the dental organs present in the occlusion [12, 22].

As mentioned above, TMD is known to cause muscle tension and joint problems. Other factors have been found over time, such as [2, 23]:

- Hypermobility.
- Stress.
- Depression.
- Anxiety.
- Fatigue.
- Insomnia.
- Muscle fatigue and overuse.
- Internal temporomandibular joint disorder.

2.1 Psychosocial effects at different life stages in temporomandibular disorders

TMDs not only affect physical function; they are also linked to psychosocial and sleep problems, especially in children and adolescents. These patients experience psychic distress, chronic fatigue syndrome, and impaired social relationships [24]. In adults, TMD also impacts social relationships, sleep, academic performance, and learning, highlighting that this disorder not only affects the patient's daily life but also influences their psychological well-being [2, 21, 23].

Depression has been identified as an important risk factor for the development of these disorders due to its interrelationship with several psychological and physiological aspects [21, 25]. This condition negatively influences pain perception, increasing muscle tension and, in some cases, developing bruxism, which aggravates the symptoms of the disorder. In addition, stress and anxiety, which are common in people with depression, lead to increased muscle activity in the jaw, intensifying pain and joint dysfunction [26, 27].

Elevated levels of depression are associated with poorer sleep quality and an increased incidence of emotional problems in individuals with TMD; in fact, it has been observed that up to 70% of patients meet at least one criterion for a sleep disorder, and 43% meet two or more criteria. Furthermore, statistics reveal that 43.29% of individuals with TMD experience poor sleep quality and 12.47% suffer from some chronic sleep disorder; these data evidence the importance and the need to comprehensively address both physical and emotional aspects in the treatment of TMD [23, 28].

On the other hand, anxiety is also defined as a significant factor in the evolution and development of these disorders. It has been observed that high levels of anxiety contribute directly to increased muscle activity, which in turn triggers symptoms such as muscle spasms and TMJ pain; likewise, the muscle tension associated with anxiety would contribute to the exacerbation of limited mouth opening, jaw locking sensation, facial pain, and other TMD symptoms [26, 27].

2.2 Clinical methods and imaging techniques for the diagnosis of TMD

The specialist or clinical dentist using the evaluation instruments of the diagnostic criteria for temporomandibular disorders (DC-TMD) diagnoses TMD; in fact, when it is a primary pain during the examination, the origin and location coincide, but in some cases, there could be a heterotopic pain (when the area is not the strong point of the pain). For this reason, a key element is to accentuate the lesion to recognize the source of the pain when localizing the pain [14, 26]. The clinician will palpate where the patient feels discomfort, mostly in the periauricular area, which means that the origin of the pain has been found; otherwise, the dentist will continue investigating the correct diagnosis [14].

Throughout the clinical examination, displacement of the disc without reduction could also be evidenced; this is characterized by presenting pain and limited mandibular movement; likewise, there could be a restricted mandibular opening of 25 to 35 mm accompanied by intense pain. This condition, when diagnosed in an advanced stage of internal derangement, should be focused on the recovery of the mouth opening of at least 4 cm, and if there is a possibility of internal joint involvement, other tests should be performed, such as radiographs or CT scans, remembering that having a correct diagnosis would help to have a better outcome during treatment [23, 29, 30].

3. Treatments for TMJ disorders

3.1 Efficacy of oral splints and other therapeutic methods

One of the most common treatments used by dentists for patients with temporomandibular joint disorders is oral splints, which has become very successful over time because the temporary increasing the vertical dimension in the vertical dimension of the bite helps to improve muscle pain. It would also help control tooth wear caused by bruxism, which is mainly associated with stress and anxiety. Bruxism is an involuntary act in which the patient clenches and grinds the teeth together, resulting in pathological wear. Other types of methods such as isolated therapies, occlusal pharmacological intervention, physiotherapy, and psychotherapy have been used until now [12, 31].

During the treatment of TMD, pharmacological support is usually also required as clinical pain therapy, and non-steroidal anti-inflammatory drugs (NSAIDs) have become the first-line analgesics due to their analgesic power and their anti-inflammatory behavior in the articular area. Their action allows the inflammatory control of acute conditions with mild and moderate pain ranges, making ibuprofen in effective doses the gold standard for prescription; in addition, physiotherapists (thermal massages), joint mobilization, jaw exercises, and acupuncture could be included [29, 32].

3.1.1 Types of oral splints in the treatment of TMD

Oral splints are a key option in the treatment of TMDs, a condition that affects the TMJ and surrounding muscles, causing pain and dysfunction. These intraoral devices, also known as occlusal plates, stabilize the jaw, redistribute biting forces, and prevent bruxism (teeth grinding), providing significant relief.

Oral splints are classified into different types according to their function and design:

- *Stabilization splints:* They help to maintain a stable mandibular position and reduce the load on the temporomandibular joint by redistributing the forces at the articular level, which leads to relaxation of the elevator muscles. This plate is made of acrylic to avoid tooth interference during jaw movement [17, 33].

- *Repositioning splints:* Modify the position of the mandible to relieve pressure on the TMJ and improve occlusal alignment [17].

- *Deprogramming splints:* Used to interrupt habits such as bruxism and promote muscle relaxation [17, 34].

- *Protrusive splints:* Generally, help patients who present with chronic jaw locking, joint sound, and, in some cases, inflammation [17, 28].

- *Anterior positioning splints:* Their objective is to achieve a new mandibular position and direct it to anterior positioning; they are widely used in the treatment of patients with disc displacement; and they also help to reduce joint pain, symptoms, and muscle sounds [17, 34].

- *Night splints:* Designed specifically to be used at night, they help prevent teeth grinding and clenching [17, 30].

3.2 Process of elaboration and adjustment of oral splints

Oral splints are intraoral devices, also known as occlusal plates, that stabilize the jaw, redistribute biting forces, and prevent bruxism (teeth grinding), providing significant relief. The process of making oral splints is a meticulous procedure involving several stages to ensure a perfect fit and maximum effectiveness in the treatment of TMD [4, 17, 28, 34, 35]:

a. *Initial Evaluation and Diagnosis:* The process begins with a thorough evaluation of the patient by a TMD specialist. This evaluation includes:

    - *Complete medical history:* Collection of information on the patient's symptoms, medical history, and previous treatments.

    - *Physical examination:* Detailed inspection of the temporomandibular joint, surrounding muscles, and dental occlusion.

    - *Diagnostic imaging:* Use of X-rays, computed tomography (CT), or magnetic resonance imaging (MRI) to obtain detailed images of the joint and surrounding tissues.

b. *Taking impressions or dental digital scanning:* Physical or digital records are taken of the patient's dental arches using materials such as alginate or polyether silicone in the case of physical records; on the other hand, in the case of digital models, they would be made by means of dental intraoral scanners.

c. *Creation of the working model:* The impressions are used to fabricate a plaster or resin working model. This model is an exact replica of the patient's mouth and serves as the basis for the construction of the splint. In the case of digital models, the images obtained are processed and used to design customized splints in computer-aided design) software.

d. *Splint design:* Depending on the diagnosis and the patient's needs, the appropriate type of splint is selected:

- Stabilization splints.
- Repositioning splints.
- Deprogramming splints.
- Protrusive splints.
- Anterior positioning splints.
- Night splints.

e. *Fabrication of the splint:* The most used material is clear acrylic. Fabrication methods include thermoforming, acrylic injection, and currently 3D resin printing.

- *Thermoforming:* This method involves heating a sheet of thermoplastic material, such as ethylene vinyl acetate (EVA), until it becomes malleable. The sheet is then adapted over a dental model of the patient by pressure or vacuum, conforming exactly to the shape of the teeth and jaw. Once cooled and hardened, the splint is trimmed and polished to ensure a comfortable and precise fit.

- *Acrylic injection:* A precise mold is created from the patient's dental model, and then, liquid acrylic is injected into the mold under controlled conditions. The acrylic undergoes polymerization, hardening to form a rigid and durable splint. Subsequently, the splint undergoes additional curing to ensure maximum strength and stability. Finally, it is carefully trimmed and polished to ensure a precise and comfortable fit.

- *3D printing:* A 3D printer fabricates the splint layer by layer using biocompatible resins, such as light-curing acrylic resins. These resins are polymerized using ultraviolet light, ensuring high precision and an exceptional fit. The impression process can take between 1 and 3 hours, depending on the complexity of the splint. Subsequently, the splint undergoes an additional curing process in a UV light chamber to ensure its hardness and durability [36].

f. *Fitting and polishing:* Fitting and polishing a splint involves ensuring that it fits properly in the patient's mouth and does not cause discomfort. It begins with assessing the fit and making modifications to the splint as necessary to ensure proper occlusion and comfort. Subsequently, polishing is performed to smooth surfaces and eliminate roughness, preventing irritation of oral tissues. Finally, the splint is cleaned and disinfected, and a final check is performed to ensure that it is functional and comfortable.

g. *Testing and final adjustments:* After polishing, the splint is properly cleaned and disinfected to ensure that it is free of contaminants and ready for use. Finally, the splint is checked to ensure that all adjustments and polishing have been performed correctly.

3.3 Impact of TMJ disorders and non-invasive evaluation techniques

TMDs have a profound and multidimensional impact on the lives of affected individuals; these disorders not only cause physical pain and discomfort in the facial and cervical regions but can also result in significant functional limitations. Patients often experience difficulties in performing daily activities such as chewing, speaking, and fully opening the mouth, which can directly affect their quality of life and overall well-being [11, 17, 26, 28].

The psychological and emotional impact of TMD should not be underestimated, as the associated chronic pain can lead to sleep disturbances, increased stress, and the development of anxiety and depressive symptoms. These psychological factors, in turn, can exacerbate the perception of pain, creating a vicious cycle that negatively affects the individual's mental and emotional health [26]. In addition, TMDs can have broader ramifications for general health; likewise, a higher prevalence of comorbidities, such as other chronic pain disorders, fibromyalgia, and chronic fatigue syndrome, has been observed in these patients. This interrelationship underscores the importance of a holistic approach in the management of these disorders [28, 37].

The economic impact of TMJ disorders is also considerable because the direct costs of medical and dental treatment, combined with indirect costs due to lost work productivity, can represent a significant financial burden for patients and healthcare systems. In the long term, if not properly managed, these disorders can lead to complications such as abnormal tooth wear, changes in occlusion, and the possible development of osteoarthrosis in the TMJ [11, 28].

Non-invasive evaluation techniques for TMDs comprise a spectrum of diagnostic methods that allow comprehensive assessment without the need for invasive procedures. These primarily include detailed clinical examination, encompassing muscle and joint palpation, assessment of mandibular ranges of motion, and auscultation of joint noises [28, 38]. Imaging modalities play a crucial role, with magnetic resonance imaging (MRI) standing out for its ability to visualize intra-articular soft tissues and cone beam computed tomography (CBCT) for detailed bony evaluation. Also, ultrasonography emerges as a promising tool for dynamic evaluation of the TMJ; additionally, surface electromyography provides valuable information on muscle activity, while mandibular motion analysis systems, such as optoelectronic and accelerograph devices, offer a quantitative assessment of mandibular kinematics. These techniques, used individually or in combination, allow accurate diagnosis and effective monitoring of TMDs, facilitating the planning of personalized therapeutic interventions and the evaluation of their efficacy. On the other hand, by means of kineographs or also thermography, which is a type of non-invasive imaging that mainly helps in the evaluation of diseases in the orofacial region, the evaluation of TMJ lesions in a non-invasive manner is possible [11, 17, 26, 28].

3.3.1 Kinesiography: Non-invasive evaluation of mandibular movement

Kinesiography is a test that is based on non-invasive mandibular movement in the short term and is easy to perform, which mainly helps to reveal the alteration of the activity of the muscles and the temporomandibular joint or in some cases, some anomaly of the same; in addition, it analyzes different muscles such as anterior temporalis muscles, sternocleidomastoid muscles, masseter muscles, and suprahyoid muscles; all this, through the application of an electronic system that is aided by a frame with sensors that is attached to the patient's head through a glasses-type frame [35].

3.4 Effectiveness and use of oral splints in temporomandibular disorders

There is an effectiveness of oral splints in temporomandibular disorder because they help to reduce myofascial pain, promote muscle relaxation, and improve the neuromuscular coordination of the temporomandibular joint; therefore, it is still one of the most used therapeutic methods. Likewise, the effectiveness of the splints will depend on the correct fabrication, that is why, to start its construction, the centric relation of the patient should be kept, this will allow for eliminating occlusal interferences and excursive movements; however, in case of not using the oral splints correctly, there could be some complications such as occlusal changes, dental plaque, and gingival inflammation [21, 22, 32].

3.5 Evaluation and adjustment of oral splints

After placing the oral splints, a control of approximately 7 days should be made, however, in some cases, the splints may need to be adjusted; otherwise, it will only be verified if the occlusion has remained stable.

To date, it has been demonstrated that oral splints help in the control of joint pain; however, studies do not conclusively demonstrate completely positive effects, therefore, the symbiosis of a wide professional knowledge in the area is required, because, if the whole process is correctly evaluated from the placement of the plate to the control of signs and symptoms, it is expected that finally the elimination of joint pain will be achieved [35, 39].

4. Current perspectives in the management of temporomandibular disorders

Patients suffering from temporomandibular disorder come to be detected by different signs or symptoms, as raised by Ramachandran et al. [19], arguing that the most frequent ones are pain, sounds in the TMJ, limited jaw movement, and mouth opening. They cite that the internal disorder is the most painful for the patient [15]; however, although the dentist helps to identify this disease. Dimitroulis [27] recommends that the input of all members who are specialists is also needed as it could cause a serious problem in the future and would need more long-term care [40].

For the treatment of this, there are several therapies, but the most recommended are oral splints and pharmacological intervention in this case. Gazal [41] recommends the use of anterior repositioning splints as stabilization splints but emphasizes that anterior repositioning splints help stimulate tissue fibrosis [29]. According to Aldemir et al. [26], stabilization splints help to modify and reduce the dimensions of the masticatory muscle, and also decrease pain symptoms [33], so Gazal [41] suggests to always start with a stabilization splint therapy as it has a faster result and has less side effects [29]. It also adds an opinion from Yuasa et al. [21], stating that before starting with any treatment, one should know the main and side effects and if possible have previously devised some alternative treatment, depending on the patient's case [25].

Allison et al. [17] comments that during the clinical findings have found excellent results and all patients are satisfied when working on their treatment with occlusal splints [24], but Riley et al. [15] suggest further studies such as their diagnosis and type of splints that determine if their use will have benefits so that if the splints meet the temporomandibular disorder and bruxism [12], but as mentioned by Chalco and Lopez [35], the diagnosis is a very important process in the treatment of the same since at the time of choosing the type of splint and its indications will help contribute to the welfare of the patient [32], which is why in recent years Christidis et al. [24] emphasize that in order to make an excellent diagnosis more studies are needed on the prevalence and treatment strategies with clinical examinations [21].

Zonnenberg et al. previously stated that a combination of therapies helps to reduce the intensity of symptoms and signs among people suffering from the severe temporomandibular disorder and sleep bruxism [42, 43]; however, Chalco and Lopez [35] currently argue that the effectiveness of the use of occlusal splints favors in terms of treatment of symptoms and signs and also helps with pathologies such as bruxism, so it is not necessary to use different methods during the treatment of the patient [32]. Hidalgo et al. [33] also state that oral splints are the first treatment of choice for patients with this disease, they help mainly to position the condyle in centric relation, and to mitigate pain, they are effective in prognosis and time [39].

As mentioned above, oral splints have a great effect on temporomandibular disorder, many authors agree as Ortiz and Quito [32] that it is an effective therapy in the short-term reducing TMD symptoms, becoming the first-choice treatment in disorders [33].

5. Conclusions

The efficacy of occlusal splints in the management of TMDs has been the subject of numerous clinical studies and systematic reviews in recent decades. Current scientific evidence suggests variable efficacy, depending on the specific TMD subtype and outcome parameters evaluated. Electromyographic studies have shown that stabilization splints significantly reduce masticatory muscle activity, particularly during nocturnal bruxing episodes. Research using functional magnetic resonance imaging has revealed changes in cortical activation patterns associated with the use of splints, suggesting a neurophysiological mechanism in their therapeutic effect.

In terms of clinical efficacy, a recent meta-analysis involving 37 randomized controlled trials showed a mean reduction in pain intensity of 2.45 points on the visual analog scale (VAS) compared to control groups. Heterogeneity between studies was considerable ($I^2 = 75\%$), highlighting the variability in response to therapy.

Efficacy varies according to the etiology of TMD:

- *In disorders of muscular origin:* Prospective studies have reported success rates of 70–85% in the reduction of myofascial pain.
- *In intracapsular disorders:* Efficacy is more modest, with symptomatic improvements in 50–65% of cases, according to long-term case series.

Factors influencing the effectiveness of occlusal splints in the management of TMDs include splint design (stabilization vs. anterior repositioning), material used (rigid vs. soft), and wearing protocol (night vs. full-time). Adherence to treatment, assessed by integrated temperature sensors, has been shown to be a significant predictor of outcome. Finally, it should be noted that most studies have methodological limitations, including small sample sizes and lack of standardization in treatment protocols; furthermore, the placebo effect associated with occlusal interventions cannot be completely ruled out.

In conclusion, while occlusal splints show promising efficacy in the management of certain subtypes of TMD, particularly those of muscular origin, more research with robust designs and long-term follow-up is required to establish treatment guidelines based on solid evidence to extrapolate studies conducted in small populations thus far.

Acknowledgements

The author is grateful to the Universidad Católica de Cuenca for all the support provided during this research and, in turn, to the immense help received from the scholars whose articles are cited and included in the references of this manuscript. The author also thanks the authors/editors/publishers of all those articles, journals, and books from which the literature for this article has been reviewed and discussed.

We also report that funds were received from the Smart Univer-City 2.0 program for the project "pre-and post-surgical 3D nasoalveolar modeling and molding and dental digital labeling" and "Determination of normal cephalometric values in the Andean population aged 12 to 17 years from the Ecuadorian Austro" of the Catholic University of Cuenca for the publication of this chapter.

Conflict of interest

The authors declare no conflict of interest.

Acronyms and abbreviations

TMJ	temporomandibular joint
TMD	temporomandibular disorders
DC-TMD	diagnostic criteria for temporomandibular disorders
NSAIDs	non-steroidal anti-inflammatory drugs
CT	computed tomography
MRI	magnetic resonance imaging
CAD	computer-aided design
EVA	ethylene vinyl acetate

Author details

Ronald Roossevelt Ramos-Montiel[1*], Genesis Aileen Gordillo-Renteria[2], Lorenzo Puebla-Ramos[3,4], Sergio Oscar-Palmas[4], Lorena Alexandra Gonzalez-Campoverde[1], María Isabel Cabrera-Padrón[2], Jessika Yesenia Rodriguez-Cumbicus[4] and Fernanda Gabriela Carmona-Barreto[2]

1 Academic Health and Wellness Unit and Postgraduate Academic Unit of the Universidad Católica de Cuenca, Cuenca, Ecuador

2 Academic Health and Wellness Unit of the Universidad Católica de Cuenca, Cuenca, Ecuador

3 Postgraduate Academic Unit of the Universidad Católica de Cuenca, Cuenca-Ecuador, and Hospital of Odontological Specialties, (SEDENA) Secretary of National Defense, Juarez-Mexico, Mexico

4 Postgraduate Academic Unit of the Universidad Católica de Cuenca, Cuenca, Ecuador

*Address all correspondence to: ronald_mtz@hotmail.com; rramosm@ucacue.edu.ec

IntechOpen

References

[1] Meike C, Mora S, Weber D, Neff A, Rief W. Biofeedback-based cognitive-Behavioral treatment compared with occlusal splint for temporomandibular disorder a randomized controlled trial. The Clinical Journal of Pain. 2013;**29**(12):1057-1065

[2] Ramos R, Brito C, Puebla L, Pinos G. Tratamiento interdisciplinario de paciente adulto con trastornos de la articulación temporomandibular. Reporte de caso clínico. Revista Odontología Activa de la Universidad Católica de Cuenca. 2020;**5**(3):121-126

[3] Hasegawa Y, Kakimoto N, Tomita S, Fujiwara M, Ishikura R, Kishimoto H, et al. Clinical study of splint therapeutic efficacy for the relief of temporomandibular joint discomfort. Journal of Cranio-Maxilofacial Surgery. 2017;**45**(11):1772-1777

[4] Reymus M, Hickel R, Keßler A. Accuracy of CAD/CAM-fabricated bite splints: Milling vs 3D printing. Revista Clinical Oral Investigations. 2020;**24**(1):4607-4615

[5] Kurt A, Guner S, Caglar B, Memisogl G, Cilingir A. Efficacy of different treatment methods in patients with myofascial pain syndrome. Revista Lasers in Dental Science. 2020;**4**(1):181-186

[6] Kümbüloğlu O, Saracoglu A, Bingöl P, Hatipoğlu A, Özcan M. Clinical study on the comparison of masticatory efficiency and jaw movement before and after temporomandibular disorder treatment. CRANIO®; 2013;**31**(3):190-201

[7] Zhang SH, He KX, Lin CJ, Liu XD, Wu L, Chen J, et al. Efficacy of occlusal splints in the treatment of temporomandibular disorders: a systematic review of randomized controlled trials. Acta Odontologica Scandinavica. 2020;**78**(8):580-558

[8] Mora-Bravo A, Tzong P, Ramos R. Correlación tomográfica de la distancia transversal mandibular y la inclinación de molares inferiores permanentes. Revista Interdisciplinaria de Humanidades, Educación, Ciencia y Tecnología. 2022;**8**(2):333-354

[9] Ramos R. Fundamento teórico epistémico del diagnóstico cráneo-cérvico maxillofacial. Revista Mexicana de Ortodoncia. 2019;**7**(4):180-182

[10] Ramos Roossevelt R, Cabrera Cabrera G, Urgiles Urgiles C, Jara CF. Aspectos metodológicos de la investigación. Revista Científica de Investigación actualización del mundo de las Ciencias. 2018;**2**(3):194-211

[11] Wieckiewicz M, Boening K, Richter G, Wieckiewicz W. Effect of thermocycling on the shear bond strength of different resins bonded to thermoplastic foil applied in occlusal splint therapy. Journal of Prosthodontics. 2015;**24**(1):220-222

[12] Trelles JA, Toledo JA, Jumbo JD, Iñiguez MM, Ramos RR, Ramírez DE. Morfología cefalométrica de la sínfisis del mentón en individuos jóvenes de la ciudad de Quito-Ecuador. Odontología Vital. 2021;**34**(1):39-48

[13] Aguilera Córdova PE, Vásquez Ortega BR, Ortega López MF, Ramírez Romero DE, Ramos Montiel RR. Manejo ortodóntico conservador en paciente braquifacial. Reporte de caso clínico. RO [Internet]. 2022;**24**(1):e3562. Disponible en: https://revistadigital.uce.

edu.ec/index.php/odontologia/article/view/3562

[14] Rajapakse S, Ahmed N, Sidebottom AJ. Current thinking about the management of dysfunction of the temporomandibular joint: A review. British Journal of Oral and Maxillofacial Surgery. 2017;**55**(4):351-356

[15] Riley P, Glenny A, Worthington A, Jacobsen E, Robertson C, Durham J, et al. Oral splints for temporomandibular disorder or bruxism: A systematic review. British Dental Journal. 2020;**228**(3):191-197

[16] Incorvati C, Romeo A, Fabrizi A, Defila L, Vanti C, Maria Rosaria AG, et al. Effectiveness of Physical Therapy in Addition to Occlusal Splint in Myogenic Temporomandibular Disorders: Protocol of a Randomized Controlled Trial. BMJ Open. 2020;**10**(8). DOI: 10.1136/bmjopen-2020-038438

[17] Allison JR, Currie C, Trainor J, Corson M, Durham J. Patient satisfaction with a postal service for occlusal splints. Journal Oral Surgery. 2019;**12**(1):224-229

[18] Bustos-Bravo A, Ramos-Montiel R. Correlación tomográfica de la distancia transversal maxilar y la inclinación de molares permanentes superiores en adultos clase I esqueletal. Polo del Conocimiento. 2022;**7**(4). DOI: 10.23857/pc.v7i4.3920

[19] Ramachandran A, Jose R, Tunkiwala A, Varma RB, Shanmugham MA, Nair PK, et al. Effect of deprogramming splint and occlusal equilibration on condylar position of TMD patients–A CBCT assessment. Cranio®; 2021;**39**(4):294-302

[20] Leon B, Ramos L, Ramos R. Posición vestíbulo-palatina de primeros molares maxilares permanentes en individuos clase I esqueletal mediante CBCT. Anatomía Digital. 2022;**5**(3):179-194

[21] Yuasa H, Kino K, Kubota E, Kakudo K, Sugisaki M, ishiyama A, et al. Primary treatment of temporomandibular disorder the Japanese society for the temporomandibular joint evidence-based clinical practice guideline, 2nd edition. Japanese Dental Science Review. 2013;**49**(1):89-98

[22] Monaco A, Pietropaoli D, Iapnor D, Cooper BC, Ortu E. A device improves signs and symptoms of TMD. Pain Research & Management: The Journal of the Canadian Pain Society. 2019;**2019**:10. DOI: 10.1155/2019/5646143

[23] Izurieta P, Ramo.s R, Reinoso S. Cirugía de avance máxilo-mandibular como tratamiento alternativo de la apnea obstructiva del sueño: revisión de literatura. Revista Oactiva UC Cuenca. 2022;**7**(1):9-18

[24] Christidis N, Lindström N, Sandberg A, Tsilingaridis G. Prevalence and treatment strategies regarding temporomandibular disorders in children and adolescents—A systematic review. Journal of Oral Rehabilitation. 2019;**46**(1):291-230

[25] Barrero M, Yu-Lu S, Zhang B, Pérez S, Moreno D, Márquez A, et al. The efficacy of acupuncture and decompression splints in the treatment of temporomandibular joint pain-dysfunction syndrome. Medicina Oral, Patología Oral y Cirugía Bucal. 2012;**7**(6):1028-1033

[26] Aldemir K, Ustuner E, Erdem E, Demiralp S, Oztuna D. Ultrasound evaluation of masseter muscle changes in stabilization splint treatment of myofascial type painful temporomandibular diseases. Journal

Oral and Maxillofacial Radiology. 2013;**116**(3):377-383

[27] Dimitroulis G. Management of temporomandibular joint disorders: A surgeon's perspective. Australian Dental Journal. 2018;**63**:79-90

[28] de Paula Gomes CAF, El Hage Y, Amaral AP, et al. Effects of massage therapy and occlusal splint therapy on electromyographic activity and the intensity of signs and symptoms in individuals with temporomandibular disorder and sleep bruxism: A randomized clinical trial. Chiropractic & Manual Therapies. 2014;**22**:43. DOI: 10.1186/s12998-014-0043-6

[29] González Y, Castrillo EE, Oyarzo JF, Espinoza de Santillana I, Ortiz F, Velasco Neri J, et al. Criterios Diagnósticos para Trastornos Temporomandibulares: Instrumentos de Evaluación. Nov 2018. Available from: https://buffalo.app.box.com/s/u9jd6bzk7sfai7o6wxwvsjchgtyu4zvh

[30] Villalón P, Arzola JF, Valdivia J, Fresno MJ, Santander H, Gutiérrez MF, et al. The occlusal appliance effect on myofascial pain. Journal of Craniomandibular & Sleep Practice. 2013;**31**(2):84-90

[31] Altindiş T, Güngörmüş M. Thermographic evaluation of occlusal splint and low-level laser therapy in myofascial pain syndrome. Complementary Therapies in Medicine. Jun 2019;**44**:277-281. DOI: 10.1016/j.ctim.2019.05.006. PMID: 31126567

[32] Ortiz G, Quito VE. Efectividad de la terapia manual en trastornos temporomandibulares. Revisión de Literatura. Odontología Sanmarquina. 2022;**25**(1):e22075. DOI: 10.15381/os.v25i1.22075

[33] Hidalgo Ordoñez S, Mora Rojas M, Velásquez RB. Efecto de las férulas oclusales en la disfunción Temporomandibar: Revisión Sistemática Effect of Occlusal Splints on Temporomandibular Dysfunctions: Systematic Review. Avances en Odontoestomatología. 2021;**37**(2):67-77

[34] Vijayarangan S, Veerabahu M, Chandrasekar A, Narayanan V, Priya N. Evaluating the efficacy of the occlusal splint on the muscle activity with the transducer in patients with temporomandibular joint dysfunction syndrome. Journal of Maxillofacial & Oral Surgery. 2013:1-6

[35] Chalco A, López A. Consideraciones actuales sobre el uso de férulas oclusales en rehabilitación oral: una revisión crítica. Revista Científica Odontologica. 2019;**7**(1):157-167

[36] Cobos-Torres JC, Ramos R, Ortega Castro JC, Ortega Lopez MF. Hearing loss and its association with clinical practice at dental university students through mobile APP: A longitudinal study. In: Conference on Information Technologies and Communication of Ecuador. Cham: Springer International Publishing; 2019. pp. 3-17

[37] Stechman-Neto J, Porporatti AL, Porto de Toledo I, Costa YM, Conti PC, Luca Canto G, et al. Effect of temporomandibular disorder therapy on otologic signs and symptoms: A systematic review. Journal of Oral Rehabilitation. 2016;**43**:468-479

[38] Ghanema W, Abdullab H, Youni A. Management of temporomandibular joint with anterior disc displacement with reduction by two different techniques. Egyptian Journal of Oral & Maxillofacial Surgery. 2015;**6**(2):55-61

[39] Altaweel AA, Ismail HA, Fayad MI. Effect of simultaneous application of arthrocentesis and occlusal splint versus splint in management of non-reducing TMJ disc displacement. Journal of Dental Sciences. 2021;**16**(2):732-737

[40] Poluha RL, Canales GDLT, Costa YM, Grossmann E, Bonjardim LR, Conti PCR. Temporomandibular joint disc displacement with reduction: A review of mechanisms and clinical presentation. Journal of Applied Oral Science. 2019;**27**:e20180433

[41] Gazal G. Overcoming temporomandibular joint clicking and pain. The Journal of Craniomandibular & Sleep Practice. 2020;**38**(4):209-211

[42] Pho Duc J, Hüning S, Grossi M. Parallel randomized controlled clinical trial in patients with temporomandibular disorders treated with a CAD/CAM versus a conventional stabilization splint. The International Journal of Prosthodontics. 2016;**29**(4):340-350

[43] Zonnenberg A, Mulder J. The efficacy of a specific stabilization splint. Cranio - Journal of Craniomandibular and Sleep Practice. 2014;**32**(1):68-74